DATE DUE

AG 1 9 '97			
SE 9 '97			
OC 5 '98			
NO 15 '99			
OC 3 '00			
NO 2 '00			
MY 30 '02			
JY 27 '04			

DEMCO 38-296

Confronting the Emotional
and Physical Challenges

PROSTATE
CANCER

Treatment & Recovery

RICHARD Y. HANDY

PB Prometheus Books

59 John Glenn Drive
Amherst, New York 14228-2197

For my Healing Presences

Return O Lord, deliver my soul
Oh save me for thy mercy's sake.
For in death there is no remembrance of thee:
in the grave who shall give thee thanks?

Psalm 6, verses 4–5

Published 1996 by Prometheus Books

Prostate Cancer: Treatment and Recovery. Copyright © 1996 by Richard Y. Handy. All rights reserved. No part of this publication may be reproduced, stored in a retrieval system, or transmitted in any form or by any means, electronic, mechanical, photocopying, recording, or otherwise, without prior written permission of the publisher, except in the case of brief quotations embodied in critical articles and reviews. Inquiries should be addressed to Prometheus Books, 59 John Glenn Drive, Amherst, New York 14228–2197, 716–691–0133. FAX: 716–691–0137.

00 99 98 97 96   5 4 3 2 1

Library of Congress Cataloging-in-Publication Data

Handy, Richard Y.
    [Male sexuality and the challenge of healing impotence]
    Prostate cancer : treatment & recovery / Richard Y. Handy.
        p.   cm.
    Originally published by Prometheus Books in 1988 under title: Male sexuality and the challenge of healing impotence
    Includes bibliographical references.
    ISBN 1–57392–074–6 (pbk.)
    1. Impotence—Psychological aspects. 2. Prostate—Cancer—Psychological aspects. 3. Male sexuality. I. Title.
RC889.H26   1996
616.6.92'0019—dc20   96–18737
                                                                   CIP

Printed in the United States of America on acid-free paper

Contents

Preface

In 1983, prostate cancer—the dreaded "ignored male disease"—unexpectedly sprang out of its dark closet to demand my life. My story is about the most personal experience a man can share: how to heal the emotional effects of cancer's threat to his life and of its cure's devastating consequence for his sense of maleness—permanent sexual impotence.

Having lived comfortably with my silent prostate for fifty-two years and knowing only that it had something to do with sex,[1] I knew nothing about prostate cancer. I had never heard it discussed. By 1988, when I finished the first edition of this book, prostate cancer remained the "ignored male disease." By then, however, I knew that:

- it had become the second most frequently diagnosed cancer in men
- more than 100,000 men would suffer its threat annually
- it was the second-leading cancer-caused death for men; after treatment, more than a third would die within five years
- little was known about its diagnosis, its recommended treatments, and the treatments' long-term survival effects[2]
- it was "curable" if treated in its early stages, but because of its high rate of recurrence, researchers defined "cure" as being symptom-free for five, ten, and fifteen years following treatment
- its "cure" produced sexual impotence in most and risked permanent incontinence in some

By 1995, when I was asked to update this book with a new preface and epilogue, prostate cancer's closet was not quite so dark; its door has been slowly opening to public view. Since the disease has become a topic to talk about in polite society, and to write about in the *Wall Street Journal,* I decided to alter this book's original euphemistic title, *Male Sexuality and the Challenge of Healing Impotence,* to acknowledge that the book is about prostate cancer and its emotional effects. The door has opened enough that we even hear about the cancerous prostates of famous men of politics, economics, religion, and sport. Dead: Menachim Begin (prime minister of Israel), François Mitterand (president of France), Steven Ross (millionaire former chairman of Time Warner), and Bobby Riggs (tennis star). Dying: Michael Milkin (junk bond king)[3] and Howard Hunter (president of the Mormon Church). Possibly recovering: Richard Riley (secretary of the U.S. Department of Education), Robert Dole (senate majority leader), and Norman Schwarzkopf (general and commander of forces in the Gulf War).

Scientific understanding of key issues about prostate cancer still eludes researchers.[4] Though more than 12,000 articles have been written about it since 1966, we still do not know what treatment, if any, to give which types of patients.[5] Since 1974 only fifteen studies on the disease appeared in mental health journals, and none of these articles is about the disease's likely emotional effects. However, since 1988, researchers have used words like "remarkable," "tumultuous," "tremendous advancement,"[6] and "revolutionary" to describe the "brave new world" that their new understandings, diagnostic technologies, and therapeutic means have created.[7] So by 1995, I had learned that:

- prostatic cancer had become the most commonly diagnosed cancer for men;[8] one of every nine to eleven American men will get the disease[9]
- of an estimated 11 million men harboring latent premalignant forms of prostate cancer, the American Cancer Society estimated that between 244,000 and 325,000 would be formally diagnosed with it in 1995,[10] a minimum of 62,000 more cases than estimated breast-cancer cases
- it remains the second-most-frequent cause of cancer-related deaths;[11] an estimated 40,400 men, or one man every thirteen minutes, will have died from it in 1995 (only 6000 fewer deaths than from breast cancer). Its death rate is increasing 2 percent to 3 percent every year[12]
- more precise chemical measures of prostate cancer's presence can now identify which patient's cancer may have escaped from the prostate or who may have posttreatment recurrence of cancer[13]
- improved surgical techniques can now reduce the frequency of impotence and incontinence[14]
- understanding of personality changes associated with prostate

cancer and its treatment is almost nonexistent, though research interest in patient well-being is now increasing[15]

However, impotence's closet door is only now inching open. The subject is currently being discussed on television talk shows. A recent television program on impotence daringly but only momentarily pictured a shadowed erection! A drug firm, Upjohn, is advertising a drug, Caverject, for treating impotence. But I know of no celebrities who have publicly talked about their "sexual dysfunction" (urologists' more acceptable term for impotence). Nor is impotence a topic of conversation among males. Erections are too close to the core of a male's identity to talk about comfortably. In cultures like the Filipino, males value their erections more than their lives—so claims one lawmaker who has proposed amputating rapists' penises as more humane than executing them. "Considering the chauvinistic attitude of most Filipino males, having one's male organ cut off is worse than death itself."[16]

Since the mid-eighties, impotence has burst out of its research closet. The explosion of researchers' interest has been, in the words of one, "staggering."[17] Between 1986 and 1992, 956 research articles were published about impotence.[18] In the hopeful words of one commentator, most of the 18 million impotent American men no longer need endure it;[19] it has become increasingly treatable.

Valuing my life more than my erections, I chose surgery that permanently made me impotent. But I had to struggle for months to heal myself of impotence's destructive emotional effects before I could come to terms with cancer's threat to my life. Remarkably, and very discouragingly, I found no guidelines, no advice, no fully honest, self-revelatory books written by other men about their hospital and posthospital experience. No one had written about how he had healed the *emotional* effects of his cancer and impotence. Researchers, in writing about the prostate and the penis, were writing as outsiders to what I was feeling. I really needed someone to write about me inside, a vulnerable person facing impotence and possible death. I have written this book, from the inside, for all of those men, and for their caring partners, who are confronted with cancer and impotence. I hope that the book will provide them the understanding that I couldn't find about how to live with and heal their despairing effects.

The words of Norman Cousins and others of the holistic medical tradition took me only partway. Focusing on how the psyche may contribute to the cure of an immediate physical hurt did not illuminate how to heal the lingering *emotional* effects of cancer's threat to my life and of impotence's threat to my maleness. The few women who had written about losing a breast to cancer showed that others felt as I did about cancer, but they also took me only partway. Losing the ability to have an erection has an impact on a man that is different from the impact on a woman of losing a breast.

My healing journey led me to see how the meanings I had attached to my sexuality had intruded into even the smallest subconscious recesses of my life. I came to understand my maleness in ways that I never had before. I found nothing written about the meanings of erections that I was discovering from my loss. Today, more men, and certainly many more women, question the prescriptive meanings of their gender. Might not what I was learning about my maleness be useful to other men, most of whom are probably as oblivious or inarticulate as I had been, about how our erections affect our images of ourselves as males and our relationships with others?

After more than a year on my healing journey, I very reluctantly began to come to terms with death and, conversely, to learn the meaning of living—the mysteries, shared by everyone, of which religion has always been the steward.

If you, my reader, elect to read my story only as a sick man's personal bout with cancer or as a middle-aged male's self-centered search to overcome the devastating effects of impotence, then my story may seem to have little value. But if you choose to discover significant insights into maleness, men's relationships with one another and with women, as well as society's overall well-being, reflected in the most personal feelings a man can share, then my story may have more enduring merit.

Having passed the physicians' ten-year marker along the road to a permanent cure, I return in the epilogue to the unanswered questions and uncertainties that I had encountered along my healing way to examine the persistent psychic effects of cancer and impotence.

By accepting my continuing search for healing, my wife has given me the support and courage to be so emotionally vulnerable. We both disclose our most intimate lives with the hope that you will also discover something of yourself, of some others, and of all persons in our story.

Richard Y. Handy
1996

Part I
The Beginning:
Three Revelations

"Doctor, I have to do something. I feel like I have one hundred pounds of dead weight pushing down on my rectum while straddling a crowbar. I can't stand for even five minutes. I can't sit. And if I lie on my back, the pain pushes up me again. You said this afternoon I could take the catheter out myself. I've got to do something to reduce this pressure."

"Okay. Take it out. Look at your catheter. It has a short end, the one that doesn't go into the bag. Cut that off with scissors. About 30cc of liquid should come out."

"What do I do about this blue thread you have stitched through the tip of my penis?"

"Cut it with scissors and then pull out the catheter. Get a urine sample in a sterile bottle so we can see what is going on inside there and can compare it later on with any changes."

"Well, thanks, doctor. I couldn't have made it over to your office tomorrow the way I am feeling at the moment."

Maryjane went downstairs to sterilize a bottle. The pain became stabbing and unbearable. Desperately I yelled, "Bring the scissors. Let's get going."

She rushed in with the scissors. I said, "Cut it here."

"No, he said to cut it here." She did. Some white drops oozed out slowly. The stabbing pain became less intense.

She was reluctant to cut the blue thread stitched into the tip of my penis, but she did. She went back to the kitchen to get the bottle. I lay back to watch this tether to the past 17 days slowly inch itself out of my mangled penis. That hated catheter; the first thing I saw when coming out of the anesthesia. I was appalled by its size. How could it be stuck up the small opening in my penis? Only later, when I began to heal, did I notice the Y-shaped slit cut into the tip of my scabbed penis. The catheter violated my most private inner self. The urine bag to which I was attached was a public reminder of my humiliation. I felt bruised, invaded, raped.

Slowly it slid out. The stabs became less and less painful. I began to feel warm, myself again. Suddenly the catheter stopped; the pain sharpened, now focused on the tender tip of my deformed penis. I didn't understand. What had gone wrong? Frantically, I yelled down to Maryjane, "Christ! Isn't that water boiling yet? How many minutes do you have to sterilize it?"

"It's supposed to take 15. Eight more to go."

All the accumulated frustration, fear, pain, and uncertainty of the past 23 days just took over. I had no patience left. I had been a brave model patient. But I had had enough. Desperately I shouted, "Come upstairs! Pull this damned thing out. I've had enough!"

She came in holding a steaming bottle with a hot pad.

"Pull it out." Before she could put the bottle down, I lost what little cool I had left. I tried to pull it. Each tug just sent sharp waves of pain through my penis. I couldn't figure out why the damned white monster refused to leave me. Half consciously, I recklessly tugged and tugged and then saw what I had not known; the catheter's tip was enlarged and it was this bulb I had to pull through the painfully sensitive tip of my wounded penis. As it slid out, a gush of energy left me. The pain flowed away; I felt very tired, not just exhausted, but numb. Some drops of urine trickled out, which we caught in the bottle.

"I want to be by myself."

Maryjane left. And for the first time I looked at my naked body. No IV, no tubes, no catheter, only a stack of gauze bandages covering an open wound draining my abdomen. My body was mine again. All mine.

I then looked at my naked penis: shriveled, wrinkled, mangled, and bare like a prepubertal boy's before his pubic hair has begun to grow. Suddenly, with no warning, out of the deepest part of myself— from where I don't know—was thrust a volcanic sob. Not tears, not a cry. Never in my 52 years had I experienced such consuming, compelling sobs, one after another. The room became black. I noticed nothing except a flickering inner darkness. I couldn't fight it. I surrendered to give voice to some inner demon, some shadowy, exploding force I had never known existed. I *became* each convulsive sob. I slipped into and out of darkness. I realized I had been denying the real meaning of my operation. That catheter had been my last tie to an absorbing, frightening, uncertain three weeks during which physical healing seemingly had proceeded right on the doctor's schedule without much help from me. But now I was on my own. I had to begin to face the real consequences of my operation: the emotional healing. The doctor said I was cured, but I knew at that moment that the healing was only just beginning. I knew it would take months.

Maryjane rushed into the room, crying in anguish, "What is it? What's the matter?"

I couldn't answer. She took me into her arms and rocked me, tearfully. The sobs had taken me over. I couldn't have stopped them even if I had wanted to. I gave up. I have never been so vulnerable. "Dearest, I . . . ," I tried to reply. I couldn't. I was at the mercy of a more powerful unknown than I had the will to stop.

Suddenly—miraculously, I later came to realize—a memory broke through my wavering darkness. So vivid, so sharp, so emotionally alive I knew it instantly. Like when one's life is relived just before impending death.

I was nine years old, lying on my back in a tub of warm water taking my evening bath. Suddenly, with no warning and for no reason, my penis started to get bigger, harder. It raised itself up to snuggle against my stomach. This had never happened before. I was amazed, awed, scared! What was wrong? I had lived with this penis and taken it for granted for nine years. What was it doing, acting like that? It wouldn't go down. I squeezed it to make it go down; it only got harder. How could I walk around with this hard thing sticking out? I became embarrassed. What would others think if they saw it? I didn't feel panicky; it just made me feel too good, warm, the way I felt when I teased a girl at school whom I thought I loved. I just lay there, watching, puzzled. My hard penis felt so good I just knew it couldn't be bad; it became my secret delightful mystery. I didn't even know words for what I was feeling: "penis," "erection," even "sex" had never been used in my family home and never would be. This left a lot of room for a vivid imagination and unselfconscious exploration later on in my teens.

This memory stopped as quickly as it had begun. I knew instantly that I was beginning to face the consequences of what I was going to have to live with: no more warm, hard erections. For the first time I felt my impotence. And I just gave way. More and more deep convulsive sobs. During one of those wavering moments of consciousness, I wondered how odd my memory was. Why had the memory of my first hard-on come back at this time of my life, 43 years later?

Maryjane kept cradling me, plaintively asking, "What's wrong? Talk to me."

I couldn't.

Then, just as mysteriously and unpredictably, another memory commandeered my mind. I was twelve. My "gang," eight boys all about the same age who knew nothing about puberty, had been fascinated for several months by the appearance of our pubic hairs. Quite proudly we would show our first hairs to one another. Poor Johnny came to mind. Long after the rest of us had moved on to explore what our lengthening penises and their erections could do, his pubic area still remained undistinguished. The warm, exciting feelings of those months of common exploration flooded back amid my continued sobs. One boy told us about a condom machine he had found in a local gas station. Someone suggested we all chip in toward the 25 cents needed to buy one. None of us knew what they were really used for, but we agreed excitedly. Since my penis was biggest when it was hard, someone suggested I put the condom on and show them how it worked. I refused.

My sobs grew deeper. I had no control or even will to flee this convulsing darkness.

And then a third memory burst out of that blackness. By this time I was able to tell Maryjane. Still sobbing, I said, "Never again will I be able to give you the present I gave you on our second Christmas together."

On that day long ago, I had told her I had a surprise for her, left the room, taken off my clothes, gotten a hard on, and tied a big red bow around it. My erections have always made me playful, and I charged into the room like a snorting bull, saying, "This is my big Christmas present just for you—always!" She blushed and hastily draped me with a nearby blanket.

Never again! That thought speared me even more deeply. I asked her to leave. I had to be alone. About 30 minutes later the sobs subsided on their own. I felt emptied. I came back to my senses, bewildered by my body's acting in such an abandoned and uncontrollable way. Like most American men, I don't cry. Even when I feel like it I can't. I have really cried only twice, and then only briefly, during 26 years of marriage. Both times I had been emotionally very vulnerable and in intense pain. I am easily moved, however, and my eyes water, though not enough for more than a few tears to inch down my cheeks. But nothing compared to what overwhelmed me today. Finally, out of that last lingering sob came an inner voice saying, *You know what you must now do.* I was not sure. Where did this voice come from and what did it mean?

I slept restlessly, waking up at 4:30 the next morning to the same inner voice telling me, *Talk. Talk your insides out. Tell your story. That is the only route to healing. You have put the last three weeks aside too long; you have neglected meanings from your past. Your memories point the way.*

Out of the darkness of that early morning was born what I called my "talking book": hundreds of hours of audio tape. It was those tapes that fathered this book. I knew I had to talk, not write. I am too controlled when I write; too self-consciously preoccupied with form, the right word. Writing gets between me and my feelings. I am livelier when I talk; it is the more direct route to what I feel and don't yet know. My healing had to be through my voice. I also knew I had to talk for me, not for others. It was I who needed to heal, not others who needed to learn. I had to be free. Free of the constraints of an ever-watchful audience. Free not to disguise or speak in euphemisms to protect .myself. Free to explore what others might revile. Free to mourn the loss of my erection and to discover what it had meant to me. Of that I was sure that dawning April morning.

1
Decisions about Unknowns and Uncertainties

I was preparing a brief that Tuesday afternoon when the telephone rang.

"Mr. Handy? Dr. Paul. Your biopsy report came back. Of the three samples I took, the lab reports one has a malignant growth."

"You mean cancer?" I asked incredulously.

"Yes."

Uncomprehending moment of silence.

"Are you sure?"

"I am going to the lab this afternoon to check the slides myself."

I remained calm, even detached. Measured and objective. I knew the pathologist had made a mistake. I couldn't have cancer. No one in my family had ever had cancer. I don't smoke. I drink only a glass of wine with dinner and an occasional beer. I don't like coffee. Not on principle; regretfully, my taste buds are descended from Puritans. I had never used drugs. I don't even like to take aspirin. I am not as straight-laced as I seem, but my enjoyments are not those that lead to cancer. Or so I thought. I practice and occasionally teach law, not an occupation especially prone to cancer—only to arrogance and contentiousness. I don't work around noxious chemicals. And I score very low on the scales that measure degree of risk for cancer or for heart disease. I have always had boundless energy. I've never even missed a day of work because of ill health or any other reason. I felt great— better than I had for several years. My spirits were high and I was looking forward to a lot of changes in the next months, for I was thinking of retiring from my firm to set up my own mediation service.

"What is the treatment for cancer?"

I didn't say "cure," not really believing there was a cure. My gut reaction was that cancer meant pain and death. Maybe that's why I ignored the warnings, though I had taken out a cancer insurance policy several years earlier.

How ignorant I was about so much. Not just about cancer, but about what my prostate did, even where it was precisely. Was it in the rectum? That is where my doctor, Tom Blake, always felt for it. What would happen if it were removed? Until the past several years, when I had had a long seige of lower back pain and intestinal upsets, my body seemed to be separate from my mind. I had seldom thought about it. I had never had trouble getting an erection. So I'd never had to learn much about what was to become the major focus of my life for months.

I should have known more, but I guess I just didn't want to. Three years earlier, Tom had found a small hard spot on my prostate and sent me to Dr. Bruce Paul, a urologist, who took a urine sample. Then, very matter-of-factly, as if this were a daily occurrence (which it probably was for him but it damn well wasn't for me), he told me to drop my pants and bend over. A gloved finger began to vigorously explore my most private self in a way it was being discovered for the first time— "massaging the prostate," it is technically called.

No one had ever gone into my rectum as forcefully before. In fact, no one else has ever been inside me there, except when Tom gently explored my prostate during my annual physical exam. My anus and rectum had never given me much pleasure, recently only pain. I've since learned a lot about the personalities of doctors and residents who examine me rectally. This kind of examination is like a personality test which tells me quite a bit about the person feeling his or her way around in there: self-confidently intrusive; gingerly tentative; shyly protective of my modesty; gently, almost lovingly, caressing; aggressively raping me with a finger of macho defiance.

The massage produced a meager drop of urine, which the micro-scopic exam showed to be infected. I had prostatitis, the cause and treatment of which remained uncertain. Dr. Paul told me to buy stock in the first company that found a reliable treatment; sales would zoom because so many men had this disease. A reassuring thought, though I momentarily wondered how I got it. From a toilet seat?

None of the drugs Dr. Paul prescribed worked but I appreciated his other prescription—that I have as much sex as possible. Maybe sex would purge the infection. This was the only recommendation I religiously and joyously tried to follow those three years! I enjoy sex and will use any excuse or try any stimulation to keep me alive. For that is what sex is to me—feeling alive.

Anyway, the nodule needed to be biopsied for malignancy. And he wanted to explore my bladder, for the only symptom I had was slightly increased frequency of urination and occasional dribbling. But since I felt fine and had no other symptoms, I went through the several days of hospitalization without apprehension. And under anesthesia I did not feel the needle penetrating the prostate or the exploration of my urinary system. I was right. No trace of cancer.

I saw Dr. Paul a year later and had another biopsy done in the outpatient operating room. Negative. Uneventful. A benign nodule. Obviously I was not the cancer type. Then Dr. Paul said he wanted to see me every six months because the nodule was not being reabsorbed. Okay. Then on one visit he wanted to do another biopsy.

My wife had stayed close by each previous time, but this was becoming routine. I went alone for my appointment, undressed and got into an even skimpier hospital gown than before. I felt so foolish and wary; it could be so unexpectedly revealing, like when I clambered onto the operating table, self-consciously holding my gown around what used to be my private parts—now very publicly known by so many. I had to spread my legs and put them on metal stirrups, much like my wife had done when giving birth to our children. No one seemed to mind. But I did! I was uncomfortably exposed.

An elderly nurse sympathetically said, "You know, there is not much dignity in this procedure." She was the only warm glow in that cold white room.

I impetuously replied, somewhat humorously, I thought, "I don't care about dignity [obviously I did], just as long as you don't find cancer."

This was the first sign of my deeply suppressed hunch that this might be *it*!

All of a sudden, and very unexpectedly, I felt a sharp pain as the doctor forcefully punched his way into me. I groaned, reflexively fought each puncture by tensing and pushing against him. I told him, "I'm fighting you. I can't help it."

I began to feel this might be for real. I asked for the first time, "What are the effects of removing my prostate?"

Dr. Paul, preoccupied with something down there, matter-of-factly replied, "Impotence and possible incontinence."

Impotence had several meanings to me. Thinking it meant I might not be able to ejaculate, I facetiously said, "Maybe I'll feel sex without an ejaculation like women do."

Silence! Not a topic to joke about. How ignorant I was. It never occurred to me that impotence meant I could never have a natural erection again. My erections meant so much to me. It was impossible to imagine life without them. I expected to leave this world at 85 still with a hard-on, maybe a little less firm and less frequently used, but capable of rising to the occasion.

When the procedure was over and I was getting back into more decent clothes, I jokingly told Dr. Paul, "You need to improve your technique. That was a lot more painful than the previous one."

"I used a different needle," he laconically replied. He later told me that I was not a typical patient. I questioned too much. Most patients just accepted his advice.

"What is the treatment for cancer?"

So began the unsought education of Rich Handy.

Impersonally, clearly, honestly, and patiently, as if he had done this hundreds of times, Dr. Paul explained that it was necessary to "stage" the cancer to see if it had metastasized before deciding on the method of treatment. I didn't quite know what "metastasize" meant, except that it was bad. I had to have a serum acid phosphatase test, which would tell if the cancer had spread, or metastasized, to other parts of my system. Then I would need a bone scan, which I also had never heard of. This would determine if the cancer had spread to my bones. I was taking notes so that I could tell Maryjane everything that evening. Only at this point did I realize that a lot more than my prostate might be involved. I began to tremble. I thought I kept my cool, taking notes. That evening while talking to Maryjane I discovered I hadn't really heard Dr. Paul clearly after all.

If the tests were negative, then I could have an operation on my abdomen to discover if the cancer had spread to my lymph nodes. If the cancer had spread beyond the prostate, then the treatment options were narrowed; taking out the prostate would not then be necessary, for the cancer would have invaded other parts of my system, creating a much more dangerous, possibly fatal, condition. I could have radiation. I had vaguely heard Dr. Paul say something about "castration" and chemotherapy. Castration? This was unbelievable. What did my balls have to do with my prostate? Might as well cut off my penis. I was not going to become an eunuch. I later learned that removing the testicles reduces the male hormone testosterone, which apparently stimulates cancer growth. Similarly, taking the female hormone estrogen could result in suppressing or even curing prostatic cancer. I wanted no part of this treatment. Fifty-two years of living with myself included having a penis, testicles, and 40 years of sexual desire. Castration and chemotheraphy would result in a Pyrrhic victory. I might live, but at what emotional cost?

If all the tests were negative—which did not mean for certain that the cancer had not spread—then I had three choices: radiation, implantation of radioactive pellets directly into the prostate, or removal of the prostate.

"How much time do I have before I must begin treatment?"

"Obviously, the sooner the better. Clinically your cancer does not seem to be that advanced; I would be uncomfortable if you postponed treatment more than six weeks. Malignancies are more aggressive and virulent in younger men such as yourself."

I had not thought of myself as young. I had recently learned I could join the Association for Retired Persons at age 55. Retirement seemed to me to mean "old." I would be a senior citizen, entitled to discounts at movies, when I was 60. And I could get Social Security at 62, only ten years away. I didn't realize how young I was to medical staff until I entered in the hospital, where everyone around me seemed to be 80 or 90. Since I considered myself older than a "young man," I thought I had time for a leisurely decision. Besides, I had too many important consultations and several scheduled court appearances I couldn't cancel.

"If we take it out, how long will I be in the hospital? How long before I can go back to work?"

"About two weeks in the hospital if all goes well. And you should be back to work a couple of weeks after that."

"A whole month? I can't drop out of my cases for a whole month."

"You don't recover from two major operations overnight."

"Two?"

"One to test your lymph glands and the other to take out your prostate."

Goddamn it, I impatiently thought, *I don't believe this is happening to me.* "I'll talk with my wife and call you back tomorrow. Thank you."

How did I feel? What did I do? Well, I didn't cry, which was the reaction of Betty Rollin, author of *First, You Cry,* to the news that she had breast cancer.[1] I never really cried the way my wife cries or some women do in my office; I only sobbed 17 days after the operation. I felt numb, cold. I didn't feel very alert. Unbelieving, I kept at my work. I pushed aside the thoughts of dying that kept intruding. How many more years did I have to live? I looked up prostate cancer in some medical books the firm kept. It was the second most frequent cancer for men, with a mortality rate of about 50 percent. Later I learned that it was the third most frequent cause of death due to cancer.[2] I squirmed when I read that the surgery resulted in one-hundred-percent impotence and a ten to twenty percent probability of incontinence. Impossible. I felt too good. I didn't feel sick, cancerous. It was only a silent microscopic clue. But when I look back at that bleak afternoon that changed so much of my life, I wonder why I remained so calm, not upset or even angry, given my fear of dying from cancer.

So I kept my cool, though once when I asked again how long I had left, I realized I had much to be thankful for. I'd lived an abundantly full life, never been bored, been my own boss, and I'd had a loving wife and two kids who couldn't be more super (if frustrating!). I had been constantly changing and learning. It is not that I dreaded dying;

I would be sad, primarily because of what my death would mean to my wife and children. Both of my parents were dead and so would thankfully be spared the anguish of losing a child. I was not ready to die, for there were too many projects I'd been working on, many close to fruition. If only I could be guaranteed six or seven more years to digest, reflect, translate, express what I had learned. I'd had many years of rich experience counseling couples separating and divorcing, people attempting through their wills to bring serene closure to their lives, or litigious persons needing healthier, less bitter ways to resolve their dilemmas and troubles. So though I still had much to live for, it wasn't as if I hadn't lived fully and happily up to that point.

I dreaded telling Maryjane. When she came home, I sat next to her on the living room couch, put my arm around her, and said, "I have cancer." Immediate tears. I remained strong, controlled, rational; Maryjane collapsed for me. I knew she was thinking of her father, who had died within months of learning of a similar cancer that had metastasized to his lymph glands. Suddenly she said, "You need to get it out *now!*" I resisted. The next weeks were critical to some of my legal cases; much of my yearly income was coming from these cases I had been working on for months. Other people's lives were involved. I had never let my clients down.

She insisted we talk to Tom, which we did that evening. He heard her worry, her fear. He asked, "Can you manage the uncertainty of not knowing for a month about how this cancer may have spread? It only takes one escaping cancer cell."

I asked, "If you had my cancer, who would you go to?"

"Dr. Paul."

I then asked, "What would you do? Wait or have it out now?"

"I guess you have to decide what is more important: your feelings of responsibility to others or the possibility that the delay might be harmful to your health."

We rephrased the question that sleepless night in bed while I held Maryjane in my arms. "If we postponed the decision even a few weeks and subsequently discovered that the cancer had spread, how would we feel not knowing if it had spread during the time we were waiting?" Phrased that way, the answer was clear.

I called Dr. Paul the next day to schedule me for an emergency bed. I dropped everything to take the diagnostic tests. I called my clients, the court, and my editor to promise I would finish by the weekend the article he had requested I write.

We urgently sought out more information. Maryjane, a librarian for a psychiatric hospital, brought home some medical books, which we read together. She was reading ahead of me. Suddenly she put her hand over a paragraph so that I could not read about the 50 percent mortality rate over a five-year period, which I later learned was a questionably high and ambiguous rate.[3] We asked a medical specialist to canvass other opinions for us. It was mildly comforting to hear him say that I had selected the most operable cancer to have! We tracked down some friends who knew of older men who had had radiation and had been satisfied with their treatment. I found no books or articles by anyone who had had cancer of the prostate and written in detail about exactly what he had gone through. Nothing like the popular books written for women with breast cancer. Provoked and frustrated by all of the uncertainties and contrasting views we dug up, we never thought of the most obvious step of going to the university's medical library and searching out the recent urological journals for articles on prostate cancer and the long-term results of different methods of treatment. Not that we would have learned much that was definite, given the lack of long-term controlled studies.

Our most emotionally painful step was to tell our children. They'd had no clue that I might be ill, for I had not told them about my biopsies. I was too vigorous and had seldom been ill, so they found this surprise difficult to believe. Lucy cried. Pete, two years younger, remained hesitantly silent, asking few questions as was his way. For the first of many times during the next weeks I was on the verge of tears. But I kept control.

The night before my hospitalization, I desperately wanted—needed— one final loving. I undressed and looked in the mirror at my erection, which still responded instantly to desire or touch, particularly Maryjane's. From somewhere inside me came a voice, *no more.* To know that our loving was to be the last of the thousands that we had had, that there would be *no more,* was too much. My erection, Old Faithful, persisted, but I could not come and Maryjane was too inwardly tearful to enjoy our last loving moment together.

I knew that in her mind the fear of my dying was ever-present. I could not ignore the possibility. We had to talk about it. I reviewed our plusses. She would have no financial worries. She was close to the children, who would stand by her. She had a network of friends who were closer to her than any friends I'd managed to hold onto. Her career was beginning to flower; she had the talents and strength to create a meaningful way of life for the years ahead. But as I reviewed our strengths, she dissolved into tears, saying how much she wished *she* had been the one with cancer.

The greatest strength we brought to the next weeks and months was our love for each other. Like all couples, we have had ups and downs and long plateaus during our 26 years together. But my work with divorcing couples has shown me that we have created an increasingly rare relationship. I know that I am not an easy person to live with, at home or at work. Lucy and Pete would be the first to say that. They've had trouble coming to terms with me. I resist accommodating, though I usually give in after first stubbornly staking out my territory. Maryjane wouldn't agree that I really give in. She says I know too many lawyer's tricks by which to make it seem like I compromise. I suppose my intense absorption in my work, which I love—the hours researching and preparing briefs, and the intensity of my emotional involvement in the lives of the men and women I counsel and defend—sometimes makes me self-absorbed. And this makes me potentially insensitive to others who are outside the periphery of my activity at the moment. So while I have filled the role of the traditional husband without ever receiving a complaint from Maryjane, I have not been the more modern companion-father to my children. They view me as more of a mystery than I am.

Just as my work is at my center, so is Maryjane's role as a mother at her center. Being more accommodative than I, the only enduring source of occasional disruptive arguments between us occurred when the children trespassed too frequently on our marital-sexual needs. I always felt she thought of me as a much better husband than father. Since being a mother was for Maryjane so consumingly primary, I as a father seemed less than adequate. For me, Maryjane and our relationship came before the children. To that she would add, "But not before your work!"

Until the children left home I suspect I was happier in our marriage than she was. Our relationship has deep roots in mutual interests and values that allow us to make consensual decisions effortlessly. When we have the information and talk it through, our decisions come easily. It is more natural for me to say, "We decided" than "I decided." Besides, Maryjane is a stubborn feminist and would never have stayed with me if I had been more authoritarian, holding all practical decisions within a secretive closed fist. We work effortlessly together as a team, collaborating on many projects. When we were newlyweds we had little money and needed a cheap place to live, so we bought a run-down old house and fixed it up together. We planned and built together a small business before I went to law school. We used to make our Christmas presents, such as bottled wine.

I am often considered too serious, even sober, conscientious, preoccupied, and not particularly sociable. But at home, I am different. I playfully tease Maryjane, snuggling up to her, kissing her on the neck, pinching, or hugging her at least ten times a day. If I neglect her she will playfully order me to hug or kiss her. We laugh a lot, primarily because of our sexual repartee. Each of us feels lonely in bed when the other is gone. We go to sleep with me shaped to her back, holding her right breast with my left hand. Because I restlessly move around in bed at night, having conditioned her to sleep on the edge, I semiconsciously move toward and away from her throughout the night. When I come back from the bathroom several times a night and crawl in next to her, she now unconsciously lifts her right breast for me to hold and squeeze. We each worry when the other is not home on time; each writes and calls and keeps track of where the other is. I have always remained faithful to her. She knows that.

Each of us dreads dying after the other. The threat of the cancer was too upsetting for us to talk about. We skimmed over it. But that threat hovered behind every decision we were forced to make in the weeks ahead. The uncertainty of the losses we were to face marshaled our energies and focused our decisions. The unspoken death of our marriage still remains unmourned. Writing this, I shudder and feel cold and heavy.

"You need to get that cancer out immediately." I knew what she was feeling. I felt her urgency too.

I feverishly worked to complete the article I'd started writing. Now I don't know how I gathered my energies to do it in the three days I had left before surgery. Half an hour after I finished it, the telephone rang. "It's time for you to come to the hospital."

So began two emotional weeks of indignities, uncertainties, decisions, discomforts, pain, and unbelief! The cancer, you see, did not seem real, since I couldn't see or feel it. It was a silent presence. I did not own any cancer. It was only a stained spot or something on a slide. My body and life were irrevocably changed as a result of what two people claimed they saw on three slides. I walked into the hospital feeling physically whole, great but potentially mortally ill. I limped out, barely able to walk and in intense pain, twelve pounds lighter, a virtual cripple for the rest of the years I had to live, but potentially cured! Emotionally, having had cancer remained a historical uncertainty for months.

Then began the interminable procession of people asking the same questions, probing the same parts: the dietician, nurses, residents, student nurses, anesthesiologists, orderlies, even a candy striper! Everyone claimed a little more of my private self. I had always been a very private person. Suddenly I felt increasingly disrobed, which I was, physically and emotionally. How fluid the boundary between me and the world around me was becoming. I felt vulnerable, even invaded, by each new caring person, particularly by those directly concerned with my anus, rectum, and penis—all of which I had spent a lifetime hiding and protecting from others. Was I to have no private self left? So I resisted undressing until I was finally ordered to do so by the nurse. It was time to be given an enema and be shaved. I hoped a male would do it; I didn't trust my reactions if one of the younger nurses had to move my too-responsive penis out of the way!

Apprehensively hovering around the edges of my consciousness, and of Maryjane's too, had been the dark uncertainty of the test results. How many more years together would they give us? Dr. Paul stuck his head into my room. The chemical tests showed no spread of the cancer. Maryjane cried as I hugged her. The suspense had been more than we knew.

Several hours later an aloof, assertive young resident whose nose reminded me of a rat's, blandly and matter-of-factly told us that the bone scan was questionable and that I needed to have x-rays taken tomorrow of my sinuses and lower spine. More uncertainty. My nagging fear exploded in a rush of angry questions directed at this unsympathetic resident—as if he were responsible! I told myself, "Handy, be careful. You are losing control." But what did he mean? Where could the cancer have spread? My sinuses? How could it have gotten to my sinuses? Where else? My lower spine? But I know I have arthritis there. "That's why you need x-rays—to confirm that."

Were some cancer cells that had escaped the prostate even now snuggling down in some warm place to multiply and kill me? I remained reasonably calm, outwardly almost rational. Maryjane regained her composure. We talked idly, skirting our uncertainties until she was told to leave. I knew how hard this was for her; we had been through so much together. The next steps I had to take alone. She left trying to hide her tears.

When a young male orderly came in to shave off my curly, bristly black pubic hair, streaked by only a few stray gray ones (I had pulled them out at first but they implacably reappeared), I finally realized the trip was for real. And I did not know where I was going, except to have my lower abdomen sliced open to explore my lymph glands.

As he shaved me clean, I saw my prepubertal self reemerging. Fortunately, my penis shriveled rather than lengthened! I was too emotionally vulnerable to have to cope with an unpredictable erection.

As I stared at my penis, I thought, "Christ, is this what they are going to make me become? A boy again? Never another orgasm. Never another erection. Never another ejaculation."

When he left, I defied those thoughts. I was going to have one more. So I showered and tried to have one more orgasm. Old Faithful erupted that last time. But it was not the memory I wanted to keep alive. But to know it was my last the rest of my life! That, I couldn't accept. It took months before I could think of myself as impotent and not wince or become mournful and nostalgic for my vigorous, impetuous cock or become angry and envious of the blue-jeaned adolescents confidently strutting down the street.

Maryjane arrived the next morning before the nurses. Mercifully, my memory of that day is blurred. Interminable x-rays of my nose and rear end, endless thermometers and blood pressure readings. Dr. Paul's second piece of good news. The bone scan was normal. A huge relief. But what would the exploratory lymphadenectomy show? Would it show that the cancer had spread from the prostate to the surrounding lymphatic system, which could then carry it to other parts of my body? The death of Maryjane's father seemed very close to us now.

I was given a shot and immodestly rolled onto a table and wheeled to the operating room, Maryjane gripping my hand as far as she was allowed to go. I got one last glance at her tearful, worried face, masked by a forced smile, doctors dressed in green getting ready, bright lights, so much busyness, so many nurses, then some barely intelligible words about something, and then nothing.

I drowsily returned to the fading afternoon light in my room. Some flowers by the window and my books that Maryjane had brought over. She was holding my hand. People coming in and out. Tubes coming out of me. An IV above me. Some other tubes from smaller bottles. An immense white catheter brazenly holding my penis up to public view. I looked at my abdomen. Shock. Disbelief. I had thought the doctor would make a small incision around my shaved pubic bone and take out a few nodes. What I saw were wire staples marching in precise order from my bellybutton down to my unrecognizable penis. My nearby appendectomy scar, inflicted on me when I was ten, was dwarfed in comparison. Unbelieving, I counted the invaders: One, two, three, four, five, six, seven, eight, nine, ten, eleven, twelve, thirteen, fourteen, fifteen, sixteen, seventeen, eighteen. *Eighteen* staples! I was dismayed. My beautiful penis publicly mutilated, no longer hidden in its protective forest; my lean proud abdomen permanently scarred, irretrievably humbled. Two yellow tubes, a Penrose drain, stuck out of a gash from which a clear, vaguely smelly fluid dripped out onto gauze bandages that needed almost constant changing. The liquid would drip down between my legs, leaving me soaked. Rather than bother the nurses, Maryjane, and later I, changed my bandages.

Thirsty, all I could have was water and a godawful liquid diet of orange juice, consommé, and cranberry juice, which made my stomach so acid that after two days I refused to drink any more. I didn't care if I died of starvation. My first act of self-assertion! It made me feel good to reclaim some control over my life.

We were tense, on edge. Had the cancer spread? What would be our choices? Dear Maryjane had sought out some information, asked for a consultation with the radiologist, contacted an outside consultant. We knew by this time that there was a large gray area surrounding the facts about the consequences of the different steps we could take. How could we send a man to the moon and create artificial hearts but not be able to tell with any reasonable certainty how long I might live if the cancer had spread? How good a cure was radiation or a radical prostatectomy that would leave me impotent and possibly with a leaky penis for the rest of my life?

Dr. Paul entered. A sharp stab went through me as I saw his face: impassive, matter-of-fact. But then he smiled. We knew! Yes, the lymph nodes were healthy. Tears came to my eyes. I didn't trust myself to look at Maryjane.

There remained that ever-present medical *but*. "But we don't know if any cancer cells have escaped." More uncertainty. One thing leads to another. A cancer cell could have escaped the prostate and not yet been picked up by any tests; it might not begin growing until a year, two, three, or more from now. I would have to be retested and examined four times a year for at least five years and even then the cancer might reappear six or ten years later. My only certainty was that my future was much more uncertain than I had ever felt it to be.

What were we to do now? We had several choices. To do nothing was unacceptable. I could have radiated pellets implanted in the prostate itself. Their long-term curative effects were not yet known, but I would remain continent and possibly potent.

Or I could have external cobalt radiation treatment, which would kill surrounding healthy cells but might not kill all of the cancer cells. It could cause urinary and rectal complications, and possibly impotence. Several years later I discovered from reviewing the research that impotence occurred in as many as 41 to 84 percent of men being treated by radiation.[4] Radiologists and urologists dispute the cure rate of radiation. Dr. Paul said that there was a 25 percent recurrence rate of cancer in those receiving radiation of the prostate. Researchers estimated that 40 percent of men who had had radiation therapy had subsequent positive biopsy readings, suggesting that they might still be at risk for cancer.[5] Though some studies reported no difference in the five-year survival rates for prostatectomies and radiation,[6] others have reported that there is a higher rate of recurrence for radiation than for surgery.[7] Ambiguity rather than clarity.

What treatments were available if cancer did recur? Because radiation kills the neighboring blood vessels and creates scar tissue, subsequent surgery would be risky because postoperative healing might be impaired. Chemotherapy and castration were then possible. And, who knows—in several years there might be more effective treatments of prostatic cancer.

Removal of the prostate meant removal of the cancer and we would know just how extensive the cancer had been and whether it might have escaped from the prostate. If cancer recurred, radiation treatment was possible. But I might become incontinent and almost certainly impotent. I couldn't go around with a drippy penis. What would I do under the stress of a trial if I started to leak? Dr. Paul said that was repairable with an artificial bladder or prosthesis. And impotence? I could get a penile implant. I was still confused about my own body. I wondered what would it be like to have an artificial erection without orgasm.

What were we to do? I knew Maryjane wanted the cancer out now. I had always feared radiology, even refusing bite-wings, much to the annoyance of my dentist. I perversely thought the dentist was just trying to pay off his x-ray machine with my five dollars. I didn't want x-rays anywhere near my balls.

We agreed we had searched out as much information as we could, so we wouldn't later regret not having done as thorough a search as we could have. Maryjane said it was my decision. But in fact it wasn't— my body was not just mine, not in our relationship. She had to live with the consequences too, particularly the uncertainty of the effects of radiation and of never having sexual relations again.

Late that afternoon on his rounds, Tom dropped in. We reviewed what we had learned and asked his advice. He said, "If it were me, I would have the cancer out now." And I felt some loyalty to Dr. Paul. He too would have it out. Of course, he was a surgeon. But I respected his judgment. He had been right about the course of the cancer and had always frankly and honestly sketched the alternatives when I pushed him.

We decided to have the prostate out. It was another one of those easy choices to make together. We did not want any cancer cells to escape during the several months of either type of radiation treatment. Radiation would serve as our insurance policy in case of future recurrence of cancer in that area. Castration and chemotherapy were impossible insurance policies. Did we consider thoughtfully the effects of incontinence and impotence? The following weeks and months revealed that we had not. But at that moment we felt good about our decision. We told Dr. Paul we were ready for the operation the next day.

The next morning I traveled the same route to the operating room. Maryjane went with me. I have no memory of the surgery. I came to late in the afternoon. More tubes, more drains, more blood pressure and temperature readings.

Then began 11 days of little wonders and occasional small miracles. And of potential self-discoveries that have taken months to realize.

About noon that fourth day, Dr. Paul told us the results of the pathological studies. No cancer found in my seminal vesicles, which I didn't know were going to be taken from me, not that I now had any use for them. But the cancer had not pierced the prostatic capsule or covering, so there was a high probability that it had not spread beyond the prostate. While there was no certainty that some cancer cells had not found their way out or that the cancer might not reappear in some other guise later in life, for all purposes he considered me cured of cancer. I felt like a farmer about to lose his way of life to a bank foreclosure, who at the last moment wins the big prize in the state lottery. The tension of the uncertainty we had suffered receded as rapidly as a tidal wave recedes after its first attack on the shore. We felt cleansed emotionally. We weren't to know for weeks that tidal waves can return.

How quickly I healed physically. Almost miraculously. Each day brought another sign of my recovery. The IV needle in my arm was taken away, then the little bottle of antibiotic or whatever it was. Sooner than I had hoped, the ward physician snipped the wire staples as I chanted: "One, two, three, . . . eighteen." Then the drain in my perineum, between my anus and the base of my penis, was pulled out. One morning the physician unceremoniously pulled out my Penrose drain a half-inch; the next day another half-inch, then another, until at the end of 11 days, he just yanked the remaining six inches out, leaving a gaping three-quarter-inch oval hole out of which continued to ooze a slimy yellowish mucus for three more weeks. The nurses became less and less interested in my temperature and blood pressure. I was taking fewer and fewer pills, though they kept me on a urine suppressant and stool softener to ease pressure on my urinary tract and rectum. Six days after walking on my own into the hospital, three days after I lost my prostate, I began to free myself from the bed. With Maryjane's help I walked to the door and back again. Each day I went a little further. Near the end of my stay I was wandering around the hospital, though still clutching my urine bag underneath my bathrobe. I was becoming free again, at least more mobile, my own person. I could even go to the toilet myself the last few days without help, though I was embarrassed that I missed the first time, not squatting right while trying to hold my urine bag at the same time.

On the tenth day since I had entered the hospital, I wanted to free myself from depending even on Maryjane, who had taken over most of the nursing care during the day. She would arrive before 7:00, bathe me, change my bandages, make up the bed, and stay with me as long as she could before she had to go to work. The tenth day, I got up at 6:30 before she came, awkwardly cleaned around my drain, gingerly washed the white stuff away from my very tender, scabbed penis, and shaved standing in front of the closet mirror. Proudly I greeted her at 7:00. Such a little step but such a big one for me to take.

The wonders of physical healing proceeded uneventfully, right on Dr. Paul's schedule, until one o'clock in the morning on my eleventh day. I awoke soaked. Everything was wet. What had I done? Most of the day before, I had sat up, typing correspondence. Had I ruptured something in my abdomen? Was fluid not being absorbed by the four-inch-square gauze bandages over my Penrose drain and so dripping down my legs onto the sheet? An hour after the nurse cleaned me up, the flooding occurred again. Now worried, I waited for the ward physician. He thought that I must have kinked my catheter, which would have caused the urine to back up into my bladder and then escape through a hole in the sutures stitching my urethra and bladder together. The urine was leaking into the perineal area and oozing out there.

Incredible and frightening. What was a hole doing in the lower part of the bladder now refashioned and stitched to my urethra? That could cause an infection, even an abcess.

A young resident accompanying the ward physician pressed my perineum and out came more urine through the drain. At least they knew. I remained vague, and still do, about how urine can seep through all of the tissues and muscles to escape out of a hole above the anus. And I remained apprehensive. Unfortunately, when the full aftereffects of this late-night adventure became manifest, I found that I'd had good reason to worry.

I slept very warily my remaining nights in the hospital. For as I physically recovered, I was resuming my restless sleeping habits. I had become catheter-shy. I wanted that catheter to remain in its proper place—actually I wanted it out.

The morning of the thirteenth day, Dr. Paul said I could leave the hospital the next day. Maryjane was ecstatic. I was relieved, worried that the midnight flooding might have postponed my departure to freedom. I hadn't told the doctors that I couldn't sit without a great deal of pain and that walking had become unfathomably more wearying. I had a hunch why but I had counted on Dr. Paul's timetable and didn't want to disrupt it.

Just two weeks before, I had strode into the hospital feeling like a whole, healthy, energetic man, but one with gnawing worries about the uncertainties ahead. Now, fourteen days later, I limped out, leaning on my wife, permanently crippled, pained by every step, wearily drained of stamina, but excitedly anticipating returning home "cured."

Driving home those twelve miles was a more emotional time for both of us than I had anticipated. Maryjane had me home again. Home has an especially personal meaning for her, and she now had me under her full care again. She was so excited she cried as we walked through the front door together. I again sensed her fear that I might have never come home. She had filled our home with an infinity of warmth and love: flowers everywhere, cleaned windows through which the early spring sun was shining, the house uncharacteristically immaculate, our bedcovers neatly pulled back, the Sunday *New York Times* on my bed, the refrigerator stocked with my favorite foods. She even had bought me a video-tape club membership so I would have movies on hand for my hours alone. Had she coaxed the white and yellow and purple crocuses to bloom and the light green haze of the trees and bushes to emerge from the gray-brown of winter just for me? Spring and hope were here.

I felt released. The ordeal seemed near its end. Driving up to the house, I noticed a lot of branches and twigs brought down by a late winter storm. I itched to get out with my power saw and cut them up. My eyes watered too when I limped through our front door. An awful lot of uncertainties had become certainties. I was on schedule. In two weeks, the doctor had promised, I would be resuming my normal life. I was released, freed; no more caring people would intrude into my personal space. And so Maryjane and I would be back in bed together where I could hold her in my arms and her right breast again—my symbol that I was on the way to recovery.

But I felt very tired. Suddenly I felt a great deal of pressure between my legs. I felt faint. I couldn't sit. Maryjane struggled to get me into bed. And all of those unformed fears and intimations that I had ruthlessly blocked from invading me during the past 14 days started to thrust themselves into my awareness.

I'd had cancer, which increased the chance of cancer in the future. I had endured two major operations. I had had my personal, private self so intrusively invaded. I did not know if I would ever again be able to control when and where I was to urinate. I would no longer have an erection or be able to enjoy sexual relations with Maryjane again. I suddenly had a very uncertain future. What to do now that I was cured physically? Get back to the business of living? Deny those emotional wounds? Let the urgencies of making a living run their natural course? But at what potential cost? I had three revelations five days later that warned me. To create too hastily superficial emotional scar-tissue could allow unknown psychic wounds to fester and even metastasize much deeper down. I risked losing the vulnerability and the will to heal emotionally as a physical wound heals, from the inside out.

Our eagerly awaited first Sunday home turned into a nightmare. Something was dreadfuly wrong. We didn't know what. Our hopes had been too high and had outrun my body's timing. I was not released after all. The hospital still had me tethered by that long umbilical white catheter hooked to my unfriendly companion—my urine bag. And then I noticed the urine was reddish. Frantically, Maryjane called the relief doctor. He seemed rather blasé and said to see Dr. Paul tomorrow.

And so began days of pain and worry. That hard lump in my perineal area was like the small speck of gravel that feels like a rock in your shoe, capturing your energy and attention with every tormenting step.

The next day Dr. Paul realized how painful it was when I cried out during his typically assertive probing of my rectum. Infection? An abscess in the lymph glands? Urine accumulated in my groin? Rupture of something? The dread postoperative consequences I had heard about had begun.

Innumerable glasses of water for more tests. Skimpy hospital gowns that no longer bothered me. What did I care now how many doctors and nurses wanted to fuss with me down there? I was safe from embarrassment. My penis had died. It had become like a shrimpy dead toenail. I felt damned low. I failed an ultrasound test because not enough liquid could be poured into my bladder to get a good picture; it was too painful. More consultations. More vile-tasting liquids to prepare me for a CAT scan. More nurses and doctors.

"Take off your clothes and put them over on the chair. We are going to shut off your catheter so we can keep liquid in your lower abdomen."

"I can't hold much without it becoming very painful."

"Do the best you can. It will take only an hour. Dr. Paul is coming to see the pictures."

My spirits drooped. An hour. The pain increased. I didn't care. I had no qualms about telling them. I was tired of being such a stoical and accommodating patient.

No word for a day. Worry. What had they found? Then Dr. Paul called. No abscess. An infection had been caused by a hole in the surgically prepared connection between the bladder and urethra through which urine could leak. More antibiotics, five debilitating hot baths a day, confinement to my bed since I couldn't walk or sit. Increasing pain.

Maryjane urged me to call Dr. Paul that dark afternoon.

"Doctor, I have to do something. The pain is too great. I feel like I have one hundred pounds of dead weight pushing down on my rectum while straddling a crowbar. I can't stand for even five minutes. I can't sit. And if I lie on my back, the pain pushes up me again. You said this afternoon I could take the catheter out myself. I've got to do something to reduce this pressure."

Then came the three memories and the beginning of my talking book. Dr. Paul's schedule—and my hope—had become a shattered promise. Physically cured, perhaps. Emotionally healed, no. My healing, growing into wholeness, had just begun.

Part II
Meditations on Healing

I had weeks—too many—to observe and muse about healing, both physical and emotional. The healing of my whole self, not just my body, was a very complicated, seemingly disorderly process. I could sense no pattern to my healing from day to day. When a weaver first threads his loom, those individual bits of colors dotted at different locations seem to make no sense. But in time, with the addition of more strands and different loom settings, inchoate figures begin to emerge and grow into definite shapes. Only when the tapestry of my healing had been completed and I had stepped back several years later to see it completely, did the intricate architecture of its patterns, their interwoven themes and feelings, become clearer and better understood.

I seek now to identify the patterns that organized my healing, that described my search for wholeness, not just to describe their individual bits of color, the tedious day-to-day changes of which they are composed. Unfortunately, my tools—words, sentences, analytic and logical skills— can deal with only one salient idea or pattern at a time, not the simultaneously occurring signs prefiguring other emerging or receding patterns. When it is completed I hope my own tapestry will faithfully portray the complex architecture of emotional healing, of becoming a more whole person.

Though Dr. Paul had pronounced me cured, I knew I was not healed. By "cured," he meant, "free of cancer." By "healed," I meant "emotionally whole." His cure took several days; mine, more than 18 months. The health professions have ignored my meaning. Seemingly, so has everyone else. I have not found any literature dealing with what

I mean by healing. Maryjane couldn't either. That has surprised me, for everyone who ever has had a major operation or—as I have seen in my practice with distraught, troubled clients—psychic pain must not only be *cured* but also *healed* if a healthier way of life or marriage or management-labor relations is to emerge.

For me, healing could not mean returning to my previous state of wholeness. It had to mean growing into a different kind of wholeness. After all, I was not the same person to whom to return. Cancer had permanently altered me and my understanding of myself and my mortality, as any serious illness or loss would. So had surgery. I was permanently impotent. Healing had to mean changing my values, my patterns of relating to others, particularly to Maryjane, and my view of who I was.

My healing progressed through certain phases, though anticipations and residuals of each occurred throughout the 18 months of my healing. I was preoccupied with physically recovering from the surgery and its immediate effects; coming to terms with my impotence and its meaning for my own maleness; struggling to accept cancer's threat to my life; and finally, emerging with a more healthy sense of wholeness.

Coming to terms with each new phase seemed to involve a similar emotional logic, most clearly seen while recovering physically: first, turning deeply inward to understand what was happening to me; second, turning outward, away from being so preoccupied with myself, to reconnect with others; third, fashioning a new pattern reconciling my past with my present state to create a new meaning for my life; and fourth, trying out that path to see if it was really the way for me. Completing each phase strengthened trust in my capacity to be my own physician and to take increasing charge of my own healing as I sought to become a more whole person.

2
Turning Inward

The loss of a sense of self

The operations had drained me of so much energy that I was quite helpless the first few days immediately following them. My consciousness became very constricted—even one-dimensional. My awareness of myself dissolved. I barely had enough energy to see the plants Maryjane had brought and the legal journals I had planned to read. Consciousness became focused on the most immediate pain, my position in bed, Maryjane's hand holding mine, the drip of the IV.

During those first postoperative days I did not feel vulnerable, since that feeling depends upon the awareness of self, of being potentially different, of having barriers, of being in opposition. I was just *there;* awareness was flat, immediate, certainly not reflective. I had no sense of personal space. If a hand came out of nowhere to thrust a thermometer at me, I reflexively opened my mouth. I did not ask why or want to know the results. I did not feel intruded upon those first days for I had no awareness of a self into which someone was prying. If infants are aware of what goes on around them but have no concurrent awareness of being a separate person, then I was like an infant, without a defined self.

The diminution of my sense of self meant that nothing was private, separate, or hidden any longer. I didn't have the energy to sustain a private self; I was so concentrated on my body that it would have been a luxury, scarcely a necessity, to protect my modesty or my dignity. The circumference of my awareness was so contracted it just did not include anything more than the immediate moment of physical recovery.

I had no sense of my individuality, no energy to even assert my will.

So all of the silent ways I had guarded myself for years suddenly slipped away, useless: my sensitivities that had warned me danger was near; my ploys and manipulative skills that deflected too-personal questions or criticisms; my intellectual coping skills, honed by years of courtroom and mediation experience, which had pleasantly put so many other people in their place. Of course these had given me great control. Now they no longer barred the massive physical and emotional onslaught that shattered my view of myself as a self-deciding, self-willing, self-controlling, and certainly, independent man.

Residuals of this one-dimensional awareness which contained no awareness of self persisted for weeks. I took my first steps on the third postoperative day. I concentrated what energy I had on taking a few steps. I knew my hospital gown was open in back, exposing my rear end. I didn't care. Three days later I did care, but not yet enough to also hide my urine bag, which I unselfconsciously paraded with me up and down the hall. Two days later I hid my companion under a bathrobe. So a measure of my healing was the increasing availability of energy to be aware of and care about how others were seeing me. I was beginning to reclaim a part of my former private, even modest, self. I began to measure my healing by how I was reconstructing myself, my individuality, my dignity. Gradually the circumference of my awareness began to expand, though I could not sustain interest in others very long without becoming very tired. I had never realized before how much energy it took to listen to other people, to be interested in what they said. As transitory as was my interest in others, it marked the beginning of my vulnerability.

Vulnerability and submission

The miracle of healing begins after a traumatic shock, such as being wounded, being told you have cancer, having two major operations in three days. The shock provokes, disrupts, tears apart the fabric of those sensitivities, ploys, and defenses unconsciously built up over the years. So though they were annihilated those first few days, fragments of myself soon began to spring back into my awareness in unpredictable ways as my energy returned. I was becoming vulnerable. I was becoming aware of how tattered my private self was, how exposed and emotionally naked I was. My penis and anus, the parts of my body I had most carefully closeted, were now open to inspection by anyone dressed in white who wanted to look at them. They were no longer protected by modesty or guarded by will. So beginning to observe how others reacted to these formerly private parts of myself spurred my awareness of myself; I became vulnerable as I began putting my private self together again.

What had been the foundation of my former self, now to be re-fashioned? I had always thought of myself as healthy, well, strong, certainly not a lying-on-my-back type of person. Not even in sexual relations. My image of myself has never had a place for weakness, pain, complaints. I had had sturdy parents, both lost in a sudden automobile accident 15 years earlier. I had never been hospitalized before, except for an appendectomy when I was ten. Emotionally, I could not believe I was flawed by cancer. I could not think of myself as possibly not controlling when and where to take a leak. There certainly was no room for the idea of impotence in my emotional image of myself as a man. I knew I was a man. I'd never had any doubts. I come across in the courtroom as a forceful, assertive, dominant male.

I have always been self-sufficient, able to take care of myself. I can cook, shop, take care of my clothes, plan, regulate time, get things done. If Maryjane is away, I do not fall apart. I think of myself as able to be independent. I can survive. I don't like being dependent.

And I am emotionally contained except with Maryjane and a few others. I have strong boundaries around myself; they protect a much more tender self. Few know how I really feel. I think this inhibition has to do mainly with my maleness, but also with my willful erections and my years of struggling to keep them hidden from others. I'm a mixture of modesties and immodesties. I have never walked around naked in front of Lucy and Pete, but often around Maryjane. I don't talk about myself much to others. I usually listen. But I can write a most immodest book like this. I enjoy sunbathing nude but dress most properly and unostentatiously in public.

For 52 years I perfected self-control, developed a very strong, assertive, sometimes overbearing will. As a consequence, I have never been one to submit willingly. I can, but when I bow my head it must be my decision. Maybe that is one reason I became a lawyer and have faithfully supported the American Civil Liberties Union. I become livid when I see others forced to bow their heads.

So how did I react to being so helpless, so vulnerable, so publicly exposed? Surprisingly, I submitted more readily than others might have thought, given my character.

I did not protest—at least initially—the hospital staff's assumption that it had a natural right to any part of my private body it wanted to peer at, touch, pinch, purge: from the cleaning lady who barged into my room without knocking while Maryjane was washing my penis, to the night nurse who demanded to see my catheter, to Dr. Paul, who just assumed I would not mind having a young resident feel for my absent prostate.

I only became aware of how readily I submitted when Maryjane asked me how I felt being examined by Dr. Paul. I had been lying flat on my back on his examination table, naked, with my legs in stirrups. There were no sheets to cover my immodesty. While explaining my case to a woman resident, they stood in front of my spread legs, observing my most private self. I noticed that she averted her eyes; that made me self-consciously aware of my total vulnerability, not just to the eyes but to whatever thoughts anyone else had. And after Dr. Paul's vigorous exploration of my prostate, I facetiously remarked, to regain some male pride, "If only I were gay, I might enjoy these examinations." Dr. Paul remained expressionless; I sensed this was not a comment, even in jest, appropriate in this situation. My wife, who had been there, was furious.

"No woman would allow herself to be so indecently exposed," she said.

Maybe that is what that nurse meant when she talked about indignity. Actually, the female nurses, quite unconsciously, I think, were much more protective of my modesty than were the males who cared for me. When changing my bandages or washing me, they discreetly covered my genitals if someone else came into the room. The male residents and physicians cared not a moment for such niceties. They were all business: objective, impersonal, get the exam done. I too began to absorb that attitude toward my anus and penis, and found that I soon was joking about what before had been unmentionable. I too had become desensitized.

What was puzzling was how readily I submitted to such "indignities," how I'd become so vulnerable, given my emotional privacy. I felt that Maryjane had overreacted. And once my penis died, it made little emotional difference any longer who wanted to see it or explore my rectum. I could no longer be aroused and my feelings could no longer be detected by changes in my penis. Not until months later, after exploring the meaning of erections and maleness, did I understand better why I had surrendered as easily as I had to the role of being a vulnerable patient.

My vulnerability was, of course, exacerbated by two major operations within three days. Since I was physically helpless, people had to do things to me to help me heal. I understood that. So, not having the energy to defy and protect, I submitted, at least initially. I became troublesome later.

Yielding is indispensable to healing, I learned. My body knew its own timing and its own needs. Just as I have had years of arguments and fights with God, refusing to submit and yield my will, and so never have been "saved," so I was constantly tempted to argue with and frequently ignore my body during those months. This probably retarded healing. Just as my attempt to resume my normal workload the ninth postoperative day may have triggered that night's urine flood, so I kept interposing my will in the way of my body's healing. One night I insisted that Maryjane allow me to wash the dishes. But I had no sooner ended my single-minded focus on getting that last pan clean than a massive pain welled up into my awareness. I had outrun my body's tolerance and had ignored what must have been many clues it had been trying to give me that it had had enough. It is said that the body does not lie. It took a long time for me to learn this. If I had yielded to Dr. Paul during that traumatic biopsy the larger needle might not have hurt so much.

So why did I finally yield my will and let my body pace my healing?

I could be vulnerable because I trusted myself and others. My body had always been very dependable, so much so that I had never been preoccupied with it until recently. For years I have worked to control my body language so that I never had to be concerned about how I was communicating to others. Courtroom work taught me to control my mouth and eyes, to modulate my voice, to sense intuitively which juror was fighting my argument and to go with his skepticism, gradually turning it around. As I have said, I could count on one hand the number of times my penis, Old Faithful, had let me down, though I had never been completely successful in mastering his moods. So I had no reason to doubt my resiliency, my inherent capacity to heal.

I could also yield because I trusted Maryjane to be my professionally suspicious advocate. Perhaps because she worked with doctors and medical literature as a psychiatric hospital librarian, she knew what questions to ask and pursue. And she was neither afraid of nor in awe of authority. Her advocacy permitted me to submit. She was not going to let anyone get away with anything she thought might hurt me. Now I know what my own clients feel when they say they will leave decisions in my hands. I am their advocate, fiercely protecting them. Just as I get angry for my clients, so Maryjane got angry for me, when anger would have eaten away my reserves—as when she learned from the ward physician after my prostate had been taken out that its removal required cutting out part of the tube through which I urinated, which subsequently had to be resewn to the bladder whose connection caused us so much concern for weeks.

"Why had we not been told this was to be done?" Maryjane demanded. "It might have changed our decision." It wouldn't have, but she was stubbornly determined to protect our right to know.

Also, I had confidence in Dr. Paul. Not just because Tom said he would go to him if he needed a prostatic operation, but because his sensitive monitoring of my prostatitis had caught the cancer in its early stages. Besides, he had been scrupulously honest in answering every question, stating his personal opinion and where others disagreed. When he was not certain, he said so. So I trusted his judgment. However, when the infection persisted for weeks, I began to question if the hole in the sutured bladder opening to the urethra was caused by careless surgery. One nagging doubt led to another. Why were his rectal exams so much more painful than those of others? Was my body telling me something when it refused to yield graciously during that last biopsy?

Monitoring my body

My body kept clamoring for attention. I became hyperaware of its every pain, discomfort. I spent prodigious amounts of energy being aware of and catering to its complaints. I was suddenly keenly aware of a bodily function that had been habitual, automatic; it became an annoying problem to solve. I could not walk for weeks without pain and the fear of fainting. One morning I "forgot" my body, hesitantly limped down the driveway to get the newspaper, and collapsed. Another morning I forgot that I had not had a bowel movement; I was outside when it began to come. I failed to get to the toilet in time. Or, on days when I tried to get along without my diaper, I would, as I had on thousands of mornings, quickly jump out of bed, only to feel warm urine leaking down my legs, flooding the sheets. If I had stopped to think, I would have rolled over on my side, picked up the bottle I kept by the bed, put my penis in it, and let the urine drip out as I gingerly inched off the edge of the bed.

I now understand why patients are so self-centered, why they want to talk about their operations, aches and pains. Healing is a naturally self-absorbing, self-centering process. It is necessary for survival to be hyperaware that one's body is no longer automatically dependable.

Such persistent preoccupation with what had been processes of living shortened my sense of perspective. I became imprisoned by each successive moment. I could not just walk up and down stairs. I had to think about each step I made. I could not just take a bath. I had to be sure Maryjane was around in case I slipped getting in and out. Little signs of healing became exaggerated moments of hope and joy, like the first time I could stop my urine for a few seconds. Little steps backward became hours of apprehension and despair, like when I could no longer sit up in bed because of that lump in my perineum.

I begin to react to my energy being so closely tethered to my body's demands with accumulating resentment, even anger. Fortunately, I had my talking book to which to vent what could have become poisoning frustrations. I learned very early in my healing that after I had talked out my feelings they did not come back to disturb my sleep. It was as if they were now outside of me because I had let them go. But my body would not let my consciousness go. For months I lamented its tyrannical grip on my energy.

Four weeks after my operation, I said:

I look at my penis and become sad. I have learned to protect its sensitive tip by pulling the foreskin over it. My scrotum is very irritated because of the urine that leaks over it into the diaper. I feel a continuous undercurrent of uncomfortableness. It is constantly pulling my consciousness back to my body, which weighs me down. I am ready to move, to soar. I am ready to get out and do things. But every time I turn around some part of my body is there absorbing an inordinate amount of my awareness. I am beginning to resent it.

Two weeks later:

Dr. Paul said today my urinary control should have come back by now. It hasn't. What is it going to be like to go back to the office or be in court and have to change my diapers every few hours? What a hassle. It takes an extraordinary amount of energy to be preoccupied about my penis, urine, its frequency, its dribbling. As soon as I stand I feel warm piss gushing out. When I walk, I feel it trickling, sometimes down my leg. I have not been able to push this leaky penis to the edge of my consciousness and get along with living. It's always in the front of my mind. I am weary. I have had enough.

The fruits of ignorance

I soon discovered that helpless vulnerability and dependency, so natural to the early days of recovery, began to interfere with my healing. As my body demanded more and more monitoring, I found I didn't know how to take care of its demands very well.

The medical model of healing is, "Trust us. We know more. Submit. Do as we say." But this left me ignorant, not able to bring my own powers as fully as I might to my own healing.

So while initially I willingly submitted my body, I soon discovered that I had yielded out of an ignorance that was to hamper and obstruct my healing for weeks. Dependency deepens ignorance, which retards healing. To become more whole, I had to educate myself. I had to tap into the power of my full mind, including, as my three revelations showed me, my intuitive subconscious and my emotional memories. But, then again, healing meant much more to me than it did to most physicians. Not once did Dr. Paul ask me about any of the themes that provoked my talking book. He had the typical physicians's view that a physical cure meant I was healed.

I guess my model of healing is, "Educate me. Knowledge, not just faith, strengthens trust. Let us work together. *I* am ill; it is not just my prostate that is diseased." Yes, my body miraculously seemed to go its own way during those 13 days of little postoperative wonders. But it certainly didn't once I left the hospital. I had to cope with a never-ending series of crises and disappointments.

My physical healing occurred in me, Rich Handy, not just in my abdomen and rectum. My feelings of apprehension and despair must have affected how rapidly I healed physically. Several years after the operation, Maryjane found an article by J. L. Marx in *Science* magazine, claiming that emotional stress affects not just susceptibility to infectious diseases but the body's immune system and capability to heal as well.[1] Healing involves the nervous system as well as the immune system. Well, I knew that first hand. My emotional reactions are my brain's way of saying it is annoyed, that something is fouling up or disrupting its efficiency. And those reactions can in turn irritate other brain connections. Later I came to know as certainly as I know I am a man that the severe stresses I had been suffering prior to my cancer must have contributed to my immune system's inability to fight off the cancer.

I guess I am too skeptical a person to accept authority on unquestioning faith. Every day in court requires skepticism. Maryjane, my advocate, was even more skeptical. So we sought knowledge to reduce the terror of the unknown, a terror whose emotional consequences blind faith would not have protected us from. Fortunately, we had a physician who, though he was a prisoner of the medical model of curing, was generously responsive to educating us. But he never initiated our education. It was not his view of what physicians did. Why else did he schedule a patient every ten minutes? Certainly not to take time to educate each one or explore anything more than their physical ailments. His receptionist was always irritated with me; my visits always lasted longer than her schedule assumed. I appreciate that many patients, like many of my own clients, want to simply be told and believe. But that faith and dependence in the long run can interfere with healing or, as with my clients, the ability to resolve future conflicts more healthily by themselves. Being a lawyer, I know full well the ambiguities involved in the issue of informed consent and the practical limitations of education. Most of us are ignorant about our bodies and the technical procedures necessary to cure us physically. But more could be done than is being done now. That was very true for me.

What was the fruit of my ignorance? Certainly, ignorance affected decisions we had to make about uncertainties that in some cases needlessly frightened and so stressed us. I've already mentioned how profoundly ignorant I was about cancer and its cure, my prostate, the physiology of my own sexuality, the scope of the operations I was to undergo, and so on. But Maryjane's and my ignorance affected my recovery by aggravating worry and anxiety and not allowing us to use our own coping resources to deal with the aftermath of the surgery. What could we have been educated about to help us avoid these stressful fruits of ignorance?

1. Just a simple diagram of my prostate, including its relation to my bladder and sexual organs, would have clarified much of our bewilderment.

2. A brief description of just what was involved in the operation on my lymph nodes and prostate would have prepared me emotionally for the shock after the operation and reduced our anger at how much violence had been done to my body.

3. Information about the nerves and muscles controlling urination would have reduced much of the worrisome apprehension I had about the incontinence. Not until a despairing month after the removal of the catheter did I learn that there were two types of nerves controlling my urinary system. And once I knew that exercising my voluntary muscles might strengthen the involuntary ones, I could work out an exercise program to help my own healing. More accurate information about the risks of incontinence (only two to four percent for skilled surgeons, I subsequently learned) would have relieved me of some anxiety.[2]

4. Demonstration of penile implants and urinary prostheses would have given us hope and made the months of depression that followed the operation much easier to live with.

5. Knowing why I was taking certain drugs and what their effects were would have reduced our apprehension. This information could have reduced my anxiety, for example, when I went for days without

having a bowel movement after I had been put on a drug to help me control my urine.

6. Information about the effect of a prostatectomy on my sexual desire and capacity for orgasm would have short-circuited so many doubts and possibly allayed my primitive fears about my maleness.

7. Knowing what to expect about a host of minor problems: catheters had bulbous ends that would cause pain when removed; commercial adult diapers were available to absorb urine once the catheter was gone; reddish-colored urine was not infrequent and not a cause for panic; yellowish mucus from the Penrose drain did not necessarily mean an infection; the gaping hole in my abdomen really would heal in time; practical steps could be taken to live with a leaky penis and to gain more conscious control over its unpredictability.

8. While knowledge is still not certain, there are cautionary steps to take that some believe may prevent recurrence of cancer in the future. At least there are books I could have read about diet, stress, and other factors to watch.

9. Knowledge about the emotional-psychological complications and aftereffects of what I experienced would have prevented much needless anxiety. Acknowledgment that there has been little, if anything, written about prostatectomies and their effects on men would have reassured me that physicians were not simply withholding information. At the very least I could have been referred to the books on the effects of mastectomies on women. The psychology is likely to be very similar, as I discovered myself only after a year of uncertain worry. Just a reading list of books by those who have reflected on their bouts with cancer would have saved me much fruitless worry. And worry is stress-inducing.

I now know how flimsy our knowledge is about many such issues. And maybe I am a stronger person for having searched out myself what is and is not known. But the fruits of ignorance have been needless pain, apprehension, too frequent dashed hopes, too much wasted energy, and retarded healing.

3
Turning Outward

The vulnerability caused by the cancer and two operations made me understand that I *was* my relationship with others, that my own identity formed a silent pattern of connections to others. I now view my illness in part as the result of disruptive and stressful relationships. Furthermore, the cancer both subtly and drastically altered my connections with others —with some temporarily, with others permanently. How could it not?

During those early days of recovery my body absorbed all of my energy, leaving little left for awareness of or interest in others. I sensed the presence of loving others, like Maryjane, but they were not really present to me as persons in their own right. As my energy returned and people kept intruding into my inner space, the circumference of my awareness began to expand. I began to note who I now was by observing how others reacted to me. I also began to become interested in others around me, like the 19-year-old boy dying of cancer in the next room; ninety-year-old Fred, restlessly walking up and down the hall, entering every room to ask for a cigarette; and the young nurse who wept when the youth next door died.

I am not quite the same person I was before I knew I had cancer. That knowledge and becoming so precipitously impotent irreversibly altered 26 years of connecting with Maryjane. It affected my relations with relatives and friends in more subtle ways.

Healing in the presence of others

If healing is to occur it must mean refashioning one's connections, not just to one's body, but to others. For what is a whole human being but a rich nexus of emotional connections to others and to invisible inner presences? Even those long dead, like one's parents, still affect one. Healing means making whole. My healing depended upon and altered my relations with many others.

So my growth into wholeness took place in the presence of healing others. But it was a shock to learn how many non-healing presences there were among my relatives and friends.

Obviously, my physical recovery was initiated by Dr. Paul and the medical staff that accompanied me along the first part of the path to wholeness. But I view Dr. Paul, the ward physician, the male residents, and even Tom to be highly competent technicians curing my prostatic cancer rather than perceptive healers healing me. They set me on the road to healing, but everyone ignored the meaning of my cancer, its possible sources, and its effects on my connectedness with others. I often wondered if it was the doctors' maleness that got in the way of their being healers. I am a male in a similar role; I am an authority figure to my clients. I too have ignored the emotional meanings of the dissolving relationships of my divorcing clients. My illness taught me that men in positions of authority have some problems. I am not judging or condemning, for we are unconscious victims of the "male" way of connecting to others.

Every male authority was detached, objective, matter-of-fact, concerned mainly with the physical. Every one was insensitive to my feelings of vulnerability, modesty, hurt, apprehension, depression. Of course, like a man, I hid such feelings anyway. I joked, kept a stiff upper lip, hid my face when tears were close, and with few exceptions kept the pain to myself and Maryjane. No one seemed to be sensitive to how I might feel when told about my symptoms or their consequences— like that brusque rat-man resident who told me about my bone-scan results. I even complained to Dr. Paul about the ward physician's lack of a healing bedside manner. No one ever asked me to share my feelings about anything, not about my reactions to the surgery, my catheter, my impotence, even about having cancer. No wonder there are so many malpractice suits these days; people think more carefully before suing someone who has cared deeply about them.

I never felt I was a *person* to any of them. That was devastating, because I needed to feel I was understood as a person whose life was now in question and certainly irreversibly altered. It was not that I wanted a psychiatrist; I knew too many from their court appearances. They were always detached, analytic, and arguing among themselves. It was not that I wanted someone to hold my hand (Maryjane could do that better then anyone else anyway) or be sympathetic or muck around in my vulnerable interior life. What I knew intuitively was that my illness was of *me,* not just of my prostate. And to not have that acknowledged and responded to appropriately created questions and doubts about how healthy my recovery was going to be. Was I to be only technically cured, not restored to wholeness? Not really a concern of modern medicine, I guess.

It was the nurses, all women, who created that climate of respect and understanding that made me feel healing was beginning, who provided me the emotional security to go with rather than against the physical healing process. Most did not pry into my personal space or intrude into my fragile defenseless self. They sensed my feelings and Maryjane's. They felt Maryjane's inner desperation the night before my second operation and brought in a portable couch so she could sleep next to me; they changed my dressings very gently; they were sensitive about my conflicts about modesty and the loss of control of my bodily functions; they accepted my childish petulance and went out of the way to demand what I had ordered when the kitchen sent the wrong meal; they recognized and encouraged my emerging desire to take more care of myself; they shared their tears over my dying neighbor, showing me they cared. I later wrote the hospital to express my appreciation for having nurses who, by responding to me as a person, helped me to heal physically as miraculously as I did.

I often wondered during those hospital days how healing can take place for those who have no loved ones around them, and what I would have done if I had left the hospital alone and had to face the subsequent complications by myself. I asked Dr. Paul about this. He said that this is one reason older people often don't want to leave the hospital;

they have no one to take care of them at home. I have already mentioned some ways that my healing took place in the presence of Maryjane. I knew she was there, even when I was plunged into nothingness by the anesthetic. To know that I was cared for so lovingly took away some pain and reduced the anxiety of not knowing what might happen if no one were there. Maryjane gave me impetus to take more active control of my own healing, though prematurely at times. Her presence surely kept my blood pressure down. These are the kinds of things that trust does.

When I got home she felt more responsible for me. I began to fret in reaction to, "Don't do this," "Don't get too tired," "Slow down," "You should try this," "Be careful." We have always argued lightheartedly about who is more dominant and bossy in our marriage. On a superficial level, I am; but she usually gets her way, for she is more often right. About my tenth week home, I told her I did not look forward to taking care of her if she became ill, for I knew she would never be as accommodating to my suggestions as I was to hers.

She quickly replied, "Well, that's because what I will want to do will be best." How could I argue with that?

We continued to work together for the many months to follow, figuring out how to cure my infection, managing my leaky penis, and occasionally cleaning up after my failure to get to the bathroom in time.

One sign of healing was reclaiming our physical connectedness again. As my energy returned I would hug her more frequently. I could not resist impetuously jumping out of bed, when I could jump without leaking, and teasingly kissing her on her neck. I still do. And she still reacts in the same way; she coyly tilts her head toward me, as if preserving her maidenly virtue, to make it more difficult for me to reach her neck. But she always thanks me. Both of us have what I can only call instinctual "skin needs" to touch and be touched, to feel physically the warmth and care of each other. Hers are even stronger than mine. I don't know what psychologists say about such needs, but for me they reaffirm my connectedness, not just to Maryjane but to Lucy and Pete as well. It was months before we could resume sleeping in the same bed, though we tried. I slept too restlessly and uncomfortably, and had to go to the john every two hours for weeks, to be able to sleep with her all night. But seven days after I got home, I woke at 4:30 in the morning and hesitantly snuck into bed with her. From then on, whoever woke up first would crawl into the other's bed for the remaining few hours each morning. That right breast needed a lot of comforting those many months before we could sleep together all night long.

Lucy had stayed with Maryjane during those first uncertain days when I was not much in this world, and both she and Pete kept in constant contact with us afterward. Lucy visited almost every week. When she knew she couldn't come, she would write. One letter that brought tears to my eyes began with, "You are the only dad I ever will have. So get well." Perhaps because it was easier for her to share her feelings of love and support than it was for Pete, I was much more vulnerable to his signs of caring. He had been enduring years of testing his maleness and any sign of tenderness or weakness was ruthlessly rejected. So when his first card signed, "Love, Pete" came in the mail and when he began to call from England every third or fourth day, I knew how deeply my illness affected his image of who he was. I remember well that fifth hospital day when he called. I was so moved, I couldn't continue the call. For the first time, I choked up and had to hang up precipitously. I was perplexed. Why would a telephone call from him make me so emotionally vulnerable that I couldn't go on? I felt so out of control. I *was* so out of control.

I had no energy to maintain any relationship on an even keel those first postoperative weeks. The cancer and my subsequent vulnerability had disrupted all of my usual ways of connecting and revealed to me feelings I had skillfully learned to ignore or put aside. Similar episodes kept repeating themselves. But eventually I recovered enough to be able to tell both children that I was able to stand on my own two feet and to save their resources for their own lives.

The presence of non-healing others

Beyond my wife and children was a much wider circumference of close and not-so-close relatives and friends. Most were elusive non-healing presences. They were too awkwardly uncomfortable about being in the presence of someone who had *cancer*, a word too painfully upsetting to use. No one ever spoke the word; it evoked too many uncomfortable feelings. Even Dr. Paul tried to sanitize it by speaking of "malignancy" and "carcinoma." I initially talked bluntly about my cancer, until I noticed how silent friends became or how uneasily they shifted the conversation to a safer topic, such as themselves. So I retreated to talk of my "illness," sufficiently vague to be safe. My cancer became like an oppressive black rain cloud against which it was best to protect oneself with an umbrella of irrelevant jokes and comments. No one could discuss the experience with me directly. Not even Lucy, who had had a lot of experience in her social work with dying people in hospices. I often felt like I was at a funeral, where we tend to talk about everything except what the mourner needs to talk about most: his feelings about the death of a loved one. All talk is circuitous and politely circumspect. Everyone, including the mourner, shares uneasily, though knowingly, in the conspiracy of silence. And of course, I quickly learned not to mention prostate. Certainly not impotence. How could they respond to that? "Oh. I am so sorry." Or, "What's impotence?" Or, "What are you and Maryjane going to do now in bed?" Or, most likely, fidgety silence, leaving it up to me to continue the conversation. Too complicated. So I became a conspirator too.

I soon became aware that I was like one of those infamous Rorschach inkblots that psychologists in court talk about. I learned a lot about my friends and relatives from the way they tried to cope with my unmentionable "illness." Years ago people didn't know how to react to someone who was divorced. Today, people don't know how to react to someone who says, "I just got out of a mental hospital," or "I have AIDS," or "I have cancer." I couldn't help it; my feelings about many people changed as a result of what I learned about them: whom I could trust; who might be present in future emergencies; who was genuinely free to care. But I have also learned to be more understanding of human frailty—I hope.

What did I learn about others? First, there are people who, from what I know of them, are so terrified of cancer and death that the only way to cope is to deny them. My older brother, for instance, never called or even sent a card. Nine months later I met him on a business trip. Before I could say anything, he said, "I hear you have been ill. Hope you're okay." Then, before I could answer, he immediately veered off as if he were fleeing for his life, and said, "I read about your divorce fight in the paper yesterday. What's going to happen?" I think of Maryjane's closest friend, who never called her those first six weeks, when she most needed some care and support to replace all that she was squandering on me. Then, feeling guilty, her friend dropped by with a box of candy and left after a perfunctory 17 minutes. A partner with whom I had worked for 18 years never called or wrote and to this day has never acknowledged my illness.

Then there were those who acknowledged the cancer but stripped it of any black implications. One friend called several times and jovially asked, "Well, how's the patient today?" When I truthfully answered, "There's been no progress," his cheerful response was, "Well, I know you're coming along fine. You sound great." In trying to reassure me, he irritated me because he was not really hearing what I was saying. I don't think I was saying, "I want your pity." I just wanted an honest acceptance of how I felt. But to him, the sun was always rising, never setting.

Then there were those who were politely dutiful. One of my four partners breezed in for three minutes, two days after my prostate operation. "The guys at the office wanted me to give you this card. We sure miss you. Don't worry about your cases. We've got them covered. I must run. I know you don't have much energy now. Take care." He never called again. Our purely professional relationship allowed no room for a personal touch or concern. It was as if he would never know how to be anything other than distantly formal and proper.

I think of Bob. I had written him that I had cancer before I knew its outcome. He drove three hours to spend an afternoon with me. I was touched by his concern, but like almost all of my friends, after his initial questions about what had happened to me, he launched into a long monologue about his new business. I had no energy to remain interested; just enough to keep my eyelids from drooping. I felt relieved when he left.

There were others, each revealing more about himself than he was aware. Harry had worked for me behind the scenes, gathering information for particularly messy cases. Maybe because of his investigative mind, I felt I was undergoing a third degree. "Where was the cancer? How did they discover it? You mean they stuck a finger up your ass? Oh, the prostate. That's got something to do with sex, doesn't it? Can you still come? What do you mean you are impotent? If you can't get a hard-on any more, what are you going to do when you get horny? You don't know whether you can get horny? Christ, man. What did you let them do that to you for? God, I'd go bananas. You can't even jerk off anymore. What are you going to do? What's Maryjane going to do? Find someone else? Ha ha." Empathic but insensitively so. But that's what made Harry a good investigator in the alleyways of divorce cases.

I understood firsthand what I have long known from my mediation work. Few people know how to really listen to others. Few know how to be *present* with someone else, particularly when the other is in distress. But because most could not listen to me, as close as I thought many were to me, I did not heal in their presence. If only they had asked me to talk about what I had gone through and what I was feeling, I would have felt they wanted to understand me.

Extending interest beyond self

One of the clearest signs of healing was the redirection of my returning energy from monitoring my own body to becoming interested in, caring about, and then seeking to reenter the inner world of others. I had never appreciated before how much energy interest, care, and love for another demand. Worry about the cancer and its consequences, forced hyperalertness to my body's undependability, and lack of energy and stamina prevented me from actively caring for and loving others. And yet I kept feeling that my healing was going to come only from growing beyond myself and reconnecting (hopefully, more healthily) to others, ultimately to love again.

My talking book is dotted with signs of this movement away from myself, though only in retrospect did I understand that that movement could only begin after I had regrounded my physical self. I needed to know and have confidence in what I could do before my energy was freed to care about others.

Four days after the operation, I began to become persistently interested in what was happening to me. I wanted to know what my temperature and blood pressure were. Why was I getting this pill? Why were they trying to suppress my bladder's function? Why this stool softener? I was moving to a different level of consciousness, requiring more energy, that enabled me to reflect back on my ongoing treatment.

The next day I was allowed to choose what to eat, a trivial but significant signal to me that I could exercise my own will again. I began to look forward to my meals, which heightened my appetite, and I became inordinately interested in each coming meal.

On my second day home, I noticed for the first time when shaving how scraggly I'd begun to look. Long hairs stuck stringily out of my neck; spotty whiskers I had missed when shaving sprouted on my cheeks. Being so preoccupied with my body's recovery, I'd had no interest in how I appeared to others. I became aware for the first time of how pale and gaunt I looked.

My body captured my energy for weeks, as the effects of the infection constantly intruded into my awareness. And as healing of the lump in my perineum inched ahead, I became more focused on my leaky, non-sexy, dead penis.

Ten weeks after the operation, I complained to the tape recorder:

I am very much aware of my penis, not because I am masturbating to try to stimulate it, but because it is so tense and weary. As my stubby, prickly pubic hairs come back in, they seem to scrape along my balls when I walk. I still feel that lump. I am feeling it now; it's painful when I push on it. This whole area has yet to heal and free my consciousness from it. I still have trouble urinating because two streams come out, going in different directions, so I miss the toilet with one of them. I have to squat down to be sure I don't miss. I am getting a vaguely erotic feeling from my daily exercises as I brace myself in the doorway and let myself fall through it, thrusting my penis out. It tells me that my body is still alive. I have to say that in this last week, my energy, concentration, and consciousness certainly have moved beyond being so focused on my body and my basic survival needs. My body is receding more and more into the periphery of awareness, since I don't have to constantly use these jars all over the house to piss. I don't have to divert as much energy into these survival processes as I have. It is a physical relief, being freed from the demands of my body. Just as it is a marvelous feeling to not have to put a diaper on when going to bed; I can now sleep nude again. Or to be able to walk around without worrying about peeing on the rugs. I feel like a caged bird that is just learning to fly—not too far for fear I might not make it. But at least it is a beginning.

But preoccupation with my penis continued to absorb much of my energy for months. The drugs that tightened my urinary sphincters had shriveled it up so much that for weeks I couldn't find it after racing to get to the john in time. That caused a number of leaky episodes as well as semi-conscious worries about what the long-term effects of my operations were going to be. My formerly manly, handsome (to me), soft four-and-a-half-inch penis had become like a baby's. I worriedly complained to Dr. Paul about its disappearance. Was this another outcome of my operation that I would have to live with? He said he did not know why that was happening, but he had heard that the penis gets smaller as one ages. Most comforting! If I had aged that much in a few months, how much of my penis would be left when I was 70? My excessive interest in parts of my body, particularly my penis, persisted for a year, until I finally accepted that this was the way it was going to be.

As more and more energy became freed from constant preoccupation with my body, I began to care more for others, particularly Maryjane. I told my recorder:

I am concerned about Maryjane's sense of well being. The operation was four weeks ago this Monday, and she has been beyond super; she has cared enormously. She let slip today she thinks of me as a child. That protective, nurturing maternal need is so strong that it can absorb her at the expense of her own full professional life. It takes time just to be with me, to put out so much energy when I am so low. The uncertainties must be affecting her. She has not had one day free of me in a month. She has not seen a friend, been away on her own, spent one evening away from me. I told her to take a day off, see a friend, go away. I will survive. She is making more comments about how busy she is, how far behind she is, how much work she has to do. So I am trying to be more cautious and careful and not make so many demands on her. I try to help with the meals; I try to sit down at the table so she won't have to bring me meals on a tray in bed. I am trying to free her from caring for me so that she will have her own time.

Several days later, I saw for the first time how worn and vulnerable she had become as a result of the trial of uncertainties we had gone through. I saw how much caring she too needed:

> She spontaneously expressed last night a strong feeling of dislike about someone with whom she works, a most rare comment for her. Then she said, "I'm trying to accommodate her to make it work." The force of that small telltale comment told me how inwardly defenseless she was becoming. At 5:32 this morning, she crept into my arms. "I am soaking wet," I said. Wearily, she replied, "I don't care." She too needed to be held and comforted. This has been a very lonely time for her, for my illness has made her realize that eventually she will be alone, that I may not be here much longer.

My care for others slowly returned, perhaps as a result of the caring others showed for me, even some of those whom I'd considered non-healing presences. I have always thought of myself as a person who cared rather than as a person to be cared for or one for whom others want to care. I knew I was more respected than loved, certainly at the firm. The reactions of my children mellowed that harsh self-appraisal. Their "Dad will take care of us" attitude, which all of us had just accepted as my paternal responsibility for 24 years, was miraculously transformed overnight into a more selfless "caring for Dad" attitude, sustained long after the immediate crisis had passed. My illness probably altered their perception of me as immortal, much as it altered my perception of them as children; I now saw that they had become caring adults.

When I first heard of the cancer, I didn't want others to know, particularly the network of people with whom I worked at the office. I felt at that time that my prostate should remain private, but have since wondered if I didn't want to discover that they didn't care about me. My cancer retaught me what I had long observed in my practice with troubled people. Few of us, particularly males, know how to care. In my occasional cynical moments, I wondered if many of us have a desire to care. A month after I had come home, a secretary at the firm got cancer of the uterus. I visited her several times in the hospital; no one from the firm had visited her. Then I remembered the plaintive but brave words of another secretary who died of leukemia ten years ago. "Rich, you are the only person who has kept visiting me, even taking the time to come to my home. Don't they care about me at the firm?" The kind of self-interest I had seen in my non-healing visitors may be the more typical human condition, whether we want to face that about ourselves or not.

It took many months before I had the energy to be able to love. Although I began to care for my clients again, calling them up and trying to listen, it took more conscious effort than came easily to me. I wasn't as freely present with them, not as understanding as I had so effortlessly been in the past. I just didn't have the energy to slip out of myself to enter as deeply into their anger or sadness or confusion as I had been able before. I was not strong enough, perhaps not as certain of myself, to abandon my self-monitoring, my lingering distrust of my own emotional resiliency. So I held back, quite unconsciously I can see now.

As close as I had become to Maryjane as a result of our trials, it was more than a year before I could trust myself and my own sexual needs and reactions to love her so that she could have some sexual fulfillment, though obviously I couldn't. But that is a more complicated story for later.

As I became more reconnected to my body and others and found ways to live with my leaky penis and limited stamina, I became less an obvious problem to myself. To others I had become my old self. I was tempted to ignore that mysterious nagging inner voice that kept hounding me each time I felt I had completed another phase of my healing. *You have more work ahead before you are healed of this cancer.*

Who was this voice?

4
The Doctor Within

Who was that inner voice that had revealed my three earlier memories and urged me to begin healing myself? Albert Schweitzer once said, "The witch doctor succeeds for the same reason all the rest of us succeed. Each patient carries his own doctor inside him. They come to us not knowing that truth. We are at our best when we give the doctor who resides within each patient a chance to go to work."[1]

That inner voice, that vague intuition, the feelings and hunches I had been having were the voice of my inner physician! Acknowledging and accepting him seemed to lead to his growing control of the course of my subsequent healing. When reviewing the course of my recovery I realized that my inner voice had begun to assert itself very early on, sometimes rudely and petulantly. Who was this mysterious inner physician I increasingly learned to trust? As I became more familiar with him over the months of my healing, I learned more about him. He certainly thought differently than I did, for he seemed to rely exclusively on hunch, intuition, intimation. His was an inner voice of wholeness, as if he had a very clear internal image of what I should become. Seemingly more at home in my dreams and unconscious, he kept giving me those miraculous intimations of the next turn I needed to take, of when it was time to change my stride, of when I was taking too big a step or when I could take a bigger one. I gradually accepted that he was my body's intuition, speaking beyond rationality and logic. I am not speaking of some disembodied spirit for which I, Rich Handy, am not responsible. The doctor is me, of course, but that part of my subconscious that sensed incompleteness, tension, beginning pain, emerging inner movements not yet in my immediate awareness or even part of my view of myself. Time and time again when talking through a problem, I would "know" when it was on the verge of being resolved, sometimes days before it actually was. True, my more consciously dominating character initially tried to take me off in different directions or at a different pace. But eventually something "warned" me that this was not the way.

My inner doctor stood for health, which is wholeness. I believe it was Carl Rogers, the founder of non-directive therapy, who wrote that each person had some inner drive to become more whole. That always perplexed me. My practical mind just couldn't make it concrete enough to know what he meant. Norman Cousins, author of *Anatomy of an Illness,* wrote of it as a very palpable, living drive to health. There were many dark moments I did not feel that inner urge to keep persisting, to keep searching for other ways to heal. When I felt like abandoning my efforts to control my urine, I remembered that Pete had written to me about a friend of his who had lost all control of his bowels due to an encounter with a land mine during the Vietnam war. Defying his physician's claim that he could never regain control of his shredded muscles, for a year he practiced tightening and releasing his anal sphincters until he won his fight. His inner doctor must have been a very persistent tyrant.

Only much later, when reading over the 653 pages of my talking book, did I appreciate how tenaciously my inner doctor had demanded that I keep searching, striving, understanding, questioning, altering my way of living and then testing that way again and again to see if it really led toward a more healthy wholeness and feeling of completeness. This all seems so abstract, elusive, almost mystical. I could, and will, reduce it to talk of my character as my ally to illustrate how I became my own doctor. But in so doing I risk becoming arrogant, someone who sees no mystery and believes his inner world is fully comprehensible —a stance I don't usually take about myself.

Character as ally

The first intimation of some guiding inner intuition of health was that fifth hospital day when I could choose for the first time what I was to eat. I did not choose the steak and frosted yellow cake I am so powerfully drawn to. Unthinkingly, I instantly chose a jello salad, chicken soup, and custard! To Maryjane a miraculous act of self-denial, given my dietary preferences. My body knew the acidic cranberry and apple juice I had been fed had violated its internal serenity, that something harsh and rich would only aggravate its sensitivity. Fortunately, I didn't have the energy to defy my body's wishes.

My inner doctor became very troublesome, even rude, on the eighth day. I had begun to monitor my own temperature and blood pressure changes to keep track of how my body was responding, and had even begun to change my own dressings in an effort to become more independent of the regular charge nurses. A student nurse who had moved in with great authority to make me her patient for the day aggressively and firmly insisted that she had to take my temperature, which the regular day nurse had just taken a few minutes before.

I said, somewhat plaintively in the presence of such authority, "It's normal. 99.0"

"How do you know? That's not normal. 98.6 is normal."

"The day nurse just took it. My body is normal at 99.0," my peeved inner doctor said. To have his word doubted!

"I have to take it."

Dutifully I submitted. It was 99. I could hear him chuckling. Then she started to put the blood pressure cuffs on me.

"It's normal, 118 over 88."

"I still have to take it." A moment later, she said triumphantly, "It's 132 over 94."

Of course, my inner doctor was beginning to fume and showing it in elevated blood pressure.

Then she suddenly threw off my bedclothes and started to lift my gown to expose my cathetered upright penis, shaven pubic area, and gauze bandages.

"I have to feel your abdomen."

"No! It doesn't need feeling," I defiantly said, pulling the cover back over my dignity.

"I have to check your bandages."

"It's not necessary. I just changed them myself."

Tense silence. She was flustered. I could see her trying to figure out what she was going to write on her chart about me. Miffed, she walked out.

Three minutes later she resolutely came back in. "If you are going to change your bandages, you must sterilize your hands first." And she proceeded to tell me how to do it in excessive detail. I smiled to myself, thinking of how all of my nurses, except one, had just casually wiped and, without "sterilizing" their hands, rebandaged me. She left. Of course she was right, but. . . .

Then the game began in earnest. Every fifteen minutes or so, she would appear with a new demand, like that it was time to change my bed, which Maryjane had done earlier. Next, it was medicine time. I said to leave it, as I had been taking it myself for several days.

"No. It is a hospital rule. Patients have to take all medicine in the presence of a nurse." I couldn't deny the reasonableness of that rule.

But my inner doctor was becoming exasperated and unkind by this time, and I blurted out, "You know—maybe you don't—I am at a different phase of the recovery process than you seem to perceive me to be." I was beginning to free myself of the definition of being a patient dependent on others, a move toward healing she was not sensitive to.

Two days later she firmly sallied into my room. "You are my patient for the day. The regular nurse is off." Aggressive care is the best nursing defense!

I winced. What was my inner doctor going to do now?

The morning started off, predictably, much like the previous one had. My inner doctor remained set, but more so. For in the intervening two days, the boundary between me and the world of those who felt they had an automatic right to my body was becoming reestablished, more firm. I had felt good exercising my will, choosing my own meals. I was extending my boundary outward, increasing my own inner space, beginning to make choices, even if they ran up against the standard operating procedures of a student nurse. One might think I was stubborn. I was. But that growth may be an essential part of healing. I had to be in touch with that inner doctor to be able to have the insight, know-how, and will to deal with all that was going to happen to me when I left the hospital. And I was discovering that I was not being trained to fend for myself. Too much nursing could get in the way of healing. I was overreacting, of course, to the message that I could not be responsible for myself.

Finally the student nurse left.

At that moment Pete called. I was very moved by his devotion. Tears came. I couldn't speak. I had to hang up on him.

A few minutes later, back she came, trespassing on a very vulnerable part of my personal space.

"Please leave. I need to be by myself right now." And I turned my back to her and retreated into what little small personal space I now had left, hiding my eyes from her, as if I had just been caught with my pants down.

A few minutes later in came another nurse I'd never seen before. Coming right up to me, staring right into my moist eyes, she abruptly said with obvious authority, "I'm the nursing administrator. How is your student nurse progressing?" What she meant, of course, was, "What's wrong with you?" I turned away to the other side of the bed; she followed me around, approaching even closer. No one other than Maryjane had ever seen me in tears. Feeling utterly vulnerable, defenseless, now conquered, I could only marshal, "I want to be by myself at this particular time, please."

Thankfully, she heard me and left. I never saw her or that student nurse again. I am not proud of myself for such troublesome rudeness. I cringe even now thinking of what my inner doctor may have done to that dedicated young nurse. I suppose patients who are obnoxiously stubborn and assert their wills in exaggerated ways violate a nurse's professional image of what she is supposed to be like. If those professional healers don't understand that a patient's assertion of his will is an indispensable step along the way to healing, to getting one's inner doctor to begin to work, they can feel rejected by their patients and retaliate with anger. But I learned I was beginning to recover. I had gotten in touch with some stubborn inner strength, something tough, hard, firm in my character that I would draw upon in the months ahead.

My inner doctor took over more and more of my healing. He demanded more technical information. He tried taking me off of drugs before Dr. Paul thought it wise and he even dared argue with Dr. Paul about the proper treatment of my inflammed lump.

"Hot baths are the best treatment for inflammations like that. I want you to take four 30-minute hot baths every day for the next two weeks."

My skeptical inner doctor agreed, until the pain seemed to get worse, not better. Then, knowing my healing mechanisms better than I could recall them, he urged me to try using cold treatments, which had helped me several years ago when heat in all forms only seemed to aggravate back spasms that had persisted for weeks. So I put cold cans of iced tea on my lower back four times a day. The first day I did it I had three miraculously huge bowel movements within the space of 20 minutes, clearing me out of several days of poisons that my stool softeners had not been able to move. But it became a contest between my inner doctor and skeptical Dr. Paul, who had never heard of such idiocy. Whether it was my inner voice or Dr. Paul's anti-inflammatory drug that eventually cured me of my lump, I don't know. The point is that my inner doctor knew intimately my idiosyncratic medical and healing history and so could point a different way that might be more in tune with my natural healing mechanisms. Norman Cousins' inner doctor must also have had a similar intuitive perception of his own healing preferences. For when Cousins learned that he had an incurable illness, his inner physician prescribed laughter as the best medicine for him, a prescription that no medical doctor could be expected to have known. Cousins recovered.

If only Dr. Paul and the nurses had made the effort to educate me so that my inner doctor could use his intuitive knowledge of my body and psyche more efficiently! If only I had been told, for example, to remember not to kink the catheter tube, which might rupture the repaired connection between the urethra and bladder. Then, knowing how restlessly I slept at night, my inner doctor could have also warned me to be more careful when I moved, which I was after that early morning flooding. But two months of retarded healing were the fruit of my inner doctor's ignorance!

Testing the inner doctor

As the infection receded, my inner doctor's insight and wisdom began to be really tested. How to "cure" my incontinence? How to live with my impotence? How to accept and transcend dying? Each question demanded persistence, the assertion of will, the nourishment of hope, the alteration of long-entrenched views of myself and my body, changes in how I was to use my body, particularly in relating to others. How fully and deeply my inner doctor knew the Rich Handy I knew and also the Rich Handy of my dreams and semiconscious life became the touchstone of my healing.

The persistent infection, Dr. Paul said, hampered curing the incontinence. Progress was so slow that by the sixth postoperative week he mentioned that I might need prescription drugs for the rest of my life. That pessimistic thought did not appeal to me at all, given my view of myself as a person not dependent on pills or other psychological crutches.

My inner doctor determined that I was not going to be one of the twenty percent who live the rest of their lives with leaky penises! It was not that I had not been heeding Dr. Paul's advice and his prescription to exercise my sphincter muscles. I had, religiously. I would lie on the floor, thrust up my buttocks, and tighten the anal sphincters while simultaneously trying to tighten my bladder muscles. Eventually I was able to do 300 of these exercises throughout the day, without creating too much pain in my groin.

It was by closely observing the subtle changes in my urination and figuring out how I could begin to inhibit its flow that I gained some confidence that I might not become a member of the 20-percent club. My first revelatory insight came while lying on Dr. Paul's examining table three days after the removal of my catheter. He asked for a urine sample. How could I give him any drops when they continuously leaked out into my soggy diaper? I was inspired (by my inner doctor?) to hold a beaker under my penis as I rose up from the table. Lo and behold, I captured a half cup of urine. I was so excited by my accomplishment that I didn't even pause to pull up my pants. Like a little boy dragging his potty proudly into the living room to show his father, I stumbled over my drooping trouser legs and hobbled into Dr. Paul's office, waving the beaker, saying, "Aren't you proud of what I was able to do?"

He wisely knew better, but smiled and said, "That's great!"

Not knowing anything about the structure of my bladder—and if it had a pocket that could store urine that emptied when I sat up— I thought at least I could catch the urine as it flowed out by gravity. That night, I held a jar under my penis every two hours when I had to get up to piss. I was dry the next morning! I told my recorder that next day:

What a remarkable feeling to have, that I can cope, that I can take a problem and solve it on my own. And I feel, "God, at least I can go through life a little more dry and find a way to adjust to my own body and hopefully in time that will lead to learning how to direct and control it a little better." I am deeply reassured that I can find a bypass strategy to deal with the messiness and uncomfortableness of those droopy, heavy wet diapers. But more fundamentally it is a reaffirmation of my ability to adapt to whatever I have to face. I had not been told anything about how to do that. I figured it out for myself. Perhaps it was figuring it out by myself that gives me confidence that I can adapt to other consequences. How many men sit home leaking, being wet, uncomfortable, feeling like little infants, not tapping into good feelings about themselves, because they have not been given the knowledge of how to control their leaky penises to some degree?

Another trivial event, but reassuring. It pointed the way that I could take to my own healing.

Five days later my inner doctor showed me the next path to take. I could get up out of bed fast enough to still have some urine dribbling into my ever-present jar. I then tried to force it out faster and found I could. The next day, I tried to stop the flow. I couldn't, but I felt the muscle respond slightly. So then I knew where the muscle was that I had to strengthen. Each time I got up from bed, I would tighten the muscle and try to speed up and slow my stream. I had many accidents that week, but I learned I could get voluntary control back over my flow. Not until I discovered that urination was controlled by two types of muscles, a voluntary and an involuntary system, did I realize how slow this process was going to be. Dr. Paul hoped that exercising the voluntary muscles would stimulate the nearby involutary sphincters.

Four days later another milestone. I began to feel the urge to urinate; up to this point, the urine just trickled out when it wished. I also discovered that after being on my feet for an hour and a half, it was time to change my diaper. My inner doctor told me to try to go in the toilet. I was able to. A quarter of a cup. But at least I was beginning to retain some urine, even when standing. Another one of those little miracles that dotted my six-month trip to continence. Not a miracle, of course, for the drug Dr. Paul had me on was beginning to have some effect.

However, my involuntary muscles were not responding as he felt they should, so he began to warn me that they might never recover. My inner doctor firmly disagreed.

I redoubled my conscious efforts. Other small miracles kept hope alive. A week later, I had the urge to urinate but when I tried, nothing happened. Were the muscles beginning to work? Two days later, I said:

Last night I went to bed with a dry diaper and woke up in the morning with a relatively dry one. As usual, I got up three or four times during the night to go to the john. I am now quite adept at stopping and starting the flow. What I discovered last night was that when I put my penis into the bottle, struggled up out of bed, and walked, holding the bottle but not trying to keep in the urine, no urine actually came out. Another small miracle? I woke up Maryjane to show her. I started my stream, then stopped it, and then relaxed my muscles. Nothing came out. Great excitement. Such a small step but it shows that the involuntary muscle is beginning to work. I can now start my stream, stop it, relax, and no urine will come out. Then I can start it again and repeat the same process. This morning I kept a bottle on my desk. When I felt the urge, I put my penis into it, walked to the john, without trying to hold in the flow, where I was able to start my stream. Hope and faith in my body are returning.

Progress inched on. Twenty days later, I wore underwear again. I had never thought putting on underwear would bring tears to my eyes. I stayed close to a john, though, and kept wearing a diaper when I was away from home. Two weeks later I drove to the A & P without wearing my diaper for the first time.

I continued to test my progress for months by slowly decreasing my dependence on the drug. Not until fully six months after the operation did I make my last comment about my leaky penis to my talking book.

The team of Dr. Paul, Maryjane, my inner doctor, and I had won the second battle. I had recovered physically and now I was cured of my incontinence. My body was effortlessly and automatically regulating itself. I was free! No more drippy penis until, as Dr. Paul laughingly warned me, I became an "old" man.

"Never," my stubborn inner doctor replied.

5
Getting Myself Together

One month behind Dr. Paul's schedule the lump had so receded from my awareness that I only occasionally felt its presence. Also, I could walk around—though I couldn't sneeze, cough, or jump—and stay reasonably dry as long as I stayed on the drug he had given me. I had begun to hope that I could at least manage physically. About this time, I began to make tentative plans for the next weeks and months. My inner physician had become quite dogmatic, telling me that I could not be healed by returning to my pre-cancer self. I had been permanently crippled sexually, subtly disconnected interpersonally, and sensitized to my mortality emotionally. Just what was I going to do about these irremediable changes? I did not expect to make a revolutionary change in my 52-year-old character; that was impossible. But I had to understand what the cancer was telling me about myself, why I had gotten it, and what I could do to prevent its recurrence. From my inner doctor's perspective, it was clear that I had to rethink my values and hopes and alter or recreate habits and attitudes. Cured, perhaps! Healed, he insisted, definitely not yet!

A beginning perspective

My emerging understanding of my illness and so of what I had to do to become more whole reflected my way of knowing and my character. For me to understand, I must first feel an idea in my gut, get my feet wet, go as deeply as I can into what my client believes is the truth. My first traumatic courtroom trial taught me more than three law courses could. To learn, I have to reflect about what I went through. In college, I had played too many academic "games"; in law school, fewer. It was more practical. Too often I just had to accept the authority of my teachers' experience, which I didn't have. So I accept that very healthy persons may not understand my view of healing. Or that those who have never had cancer may not understand its silent terror. Or that women may not understand why the loss of an erection can be devastating.

Reading my day-to-day recorded meditations several years later only sensitized me further to how my character and my illness had been so inextricably intertwined and why my search for wholeness had to take the direction that it had. My ongoing day-to-day experience was messily kaleidoscopic, repetitious, exaggerated, seemingly unordered, directionless, even miraculous, until seen in retrospect. But reimmersing myself in the details of how I had regained urinary control, for example, had the virtue of keeping the whole complex picture vividly in mind. My kind of mind probably inclined me toward viewing illness more holistically, contextually. I remember a professor trying to explain why I had so much difficulty understanding psychology. "Rich," he exasperatedly said one day, "stop asking, 'Where is the person?' so much. Scientists have to break up persons into habits, memories, and drives to be able to study them in the laboratory." I decided then that I had the soul of a poet and so majored in English.

Not surprisingly then, my experienced-based "contextual" mind responded to Norman Cousins' tale of how he cured himself of a diagnosed fatal illness by self-healing laughter and subsequently "cured" himself of a cardiac insufficiency by vigorous exercise. Commenting on the thousands of letters he had received from physicians, Cousins wrote:

> [they] have demolished any notion that physicians are universally resistant to psychological, moral, or spiritual factors in the healing process. Most doctors recognize that medicine is just as much an art as it is a science and that the most important knowledge in medicine to be learned or taught is the way the human mind and body can summon innermost resources to meet extraordinary challenges.[1]

What compelled me to take a much broader view of my illness were my inner physician's "miracles." My legal training had taught me something of the rules of evidence. Events that occur contiguously in time are, for example, not necessarily causally related. What I felt were little "miracles" might well be dismissed by scientists as too feeble "evidence" on which to construct a view of an illness. My skeptical legal mind would agree. But since I acted on the basis of such intuitions and drew ideas from seemingly miraculous coincidences—though they probably seemed silly and mystical to Dr. Paul or other more objective observers—the resulting perspective became true for me.

Knowing how skeptical I was, my inner physician ingeniously prepared me to be more receptive to his ministry by shocking and provoking me with "miracles." In retrospect, I now see that the first three revelations, which so dramatically prefigured the course of my subsequent healing, had the same effect that Jesus' "miracles" had on the disbelievers of his day. They caught my attention; shook, puzzled, and provoked my resistant mind; made me more open, receptive, eventually even trusting. I was converted into a believer in and a follower of my inner doctor.

Most of my healing "miracles" were what I called "miraculous coincidences." One type was the frequency with which a symptom or pain disappeared after I had talked about its meaning to the tape recorder. It was as if by talking I expelled the poison from my system. For example, five weeks after my operation, I was feeling very dreary, having expected to be back to work by this time. The infectious pain persisted and was no better, even though Dr. Paul claimed that the prostatic area, where the pain was localized, was healing "nicely." I was in a morbid, black mood that turned me more deeply inward than I had been for some time. Many doubts and hurts poured out when I talked. The next morning the pain had become much less intense. I was able to sit for the first time by putting a telephone book under each thigh, leaving a space between so no pressure was put on the perineal area. I had been unable to do this the day before. A quantum leap in healing!

These miracles taught me how systemic is the process of healing. Healing involves far more than just the physical-biological-medical approach. For me healing obviously involved my emotions, character, and values. Out of my more primitive psyche would unexpectedly burst an intimation, a prefiguration, that became reality the next day or, as with the revelations, months later. As the infection slowly receded,

I became increasingly preoccupied with my incontinence. As hints appeared that I could live with it, thoughts about my impotence erratically began to occur. As I learned to live with my dead penis, I began to feel I had the strength to enter more deeply into the meaning of my cancer and dying. Weeks before nearing the end of this phase of healing, more and more glimmers that my trip was almost completed began to light up my path.

Character as a hindrance to healing

My inner doctor gave me many hints that my healing was not independent of my character, particularly when I seemed to fight and resist his guidance. Only when I began to appreciate his efforts did I begin to understand that my character could also be an ally to my healing.

As healing progressed, I became increasingly aware of how my character undermined it, and eventually of how it may even have contributed to my illness. The early hospital days and routines, combined with my physical vulnerability and lack of energy, muted my character's effects. But as my healing moved from the almost automatic physical-psychic to the arduously fashioned psychic-physical, my character became provokingly troublesome to my well-being. Because most physicians don't follow their patients into their homes, where their ways of coping with their illness become more transparent, they may not see clearly how character affects healing. The consequence is that surgeons may ignore how a patient's character may be both an enemy and friend to their efforts.

How did my character hinder my recovery?

• By scrupulous conscientiousness to my clients: "Doctor, can I postpone treatment until late spring, when I will have completed some important cases?" As the infection and pain dragged on, I became increasingly itchy and tense about not being available for other clients whom I had not notified of my illness. I had planned on only a month of incapacity. Effects? Apprehension and guilt.

• By driving ahead to complete unfinished business: Five days after my prostatectomy, I had my office set up around my bed, including stacks of legal journals on the window shelf, files of correspondence, some unfinished briefs, my typewriter, a radio to mask the bustling noises of the hospital that undermined my fragile ability to concentrate, a sign on the door, "Please do not disturb." Effects? Possible rupture of the bladder-urethra connection, which led to infection. Denial of the significance of cancer and the necessity to alter my way of life.

• By a single-minded concentration that shut out my body's distress: I got so wrapped up in a book, I did not notice the accumulating pain resulting from prolonged lying in one position. Concentrating on doing the dishes made me almost faint from the emergent pain. Effect? Heightened strain on my body.

• By impatience with most everything: "How long will I be hospitalized?" "When can I go home?" "Why is this damned lump not going away?" "I've had 37 half-hour hot baths. It's no better." Six weeks, ten weeks, eighteen weeks after the operation, "Will I ever be able to stay dry on my own, without leaking, suffering cold, wet diapers, dribbling when I cough?" Effects? Deepening depression. Increased irritability sporadically directed toward Maryjane.

• By outpacing my available energy resources almost every day: I emotionally collapsed for two days after my first half day back at the office. Effects? Physical exhaustion and aggravation of incontinence.

• By frugality: "Doctor, why does this cost so much?" Fury that Blue Cross had to pay such an uncomprehendingly exorbitant hospital bill of $18,535; $1790 for drugs alone. I was apoplectic that occupational therapy charged $81.50 for an Incentive Spirometer, essentially a bag to blow into to exercise one's lungs, which I used only three times, which was never monitored, and which I left behind for the next patient to use, probably to be charged $81.50 also. Effects? Heightened blood pressure. Lingering anger, even now, five years later, but more sensitivity to my own clients' reactions to my bills!

• By suppressed emotional reactions: I was unable to cry, become angry, or be anything other than controlled and reasonably calm. Outwardly, I was an accepting, model patient. Effects? Increasing moodiness and pessimism with growing expectation of recurrence of cancer. Sapping will to heal. Bouts of resignation and defeat.

So my irritating character got in the way of healing.

It also spurred me to take more active command of my healing.

"Why me?"

My healing was led by my curious, questioning mind. Why? Why is healing so slow? What if we try this? Why didn't that work? Why did I get cancer? What can I do to prevent its recurrence? Why? Why? Why? These *whys* came to a head about seven weeks after the operation when I began to see the light beyond the daily gray clouds and sought out answers to some of the whys.

Constantly hovering in my mind's black background was the fact that cancer of the prostate, lung, breast, and colon were the four major cancer killers. I had earlier read that of the 100,000 men who got prostatic cancer each year, 50 percent were still alive five years later. Much later I read that the survival rate was improving. Depending upon the severity of the cancer, from 75 to 85 percent might still be alive five years later.[2] Five years was a very short time to my way of thinking. What about ten, even fifteen, years? Was twenty too much to hope for? Persons who have had cancer and who survived the magical five year criterion of "cure" are now known to average lower survival rates ten and fifteen years later than persons who have never had cancer. Since there is no way to tell if cancer still remains in a person, there is no way to tell who will and will not survive even five years, let alone the twenty I would settle for.[3] What was most troubling was the continuing uncertainty and meaning of such figures. Seeming "advances" in curing cancer can be deceptive for they may be primarily the result of diagnosing and treating cancer earlier, rather than of increasing efficacy of treatment.[4] Most sobering was a *Science 84* summary of what was known about cure rates, which Maryjane reluctantly showed me, fortunately after I had also considered myself healed; before it might have deepened my pessimism:

> Why is cancer really so hard to cure? . . . Most potentially fatal human cancers eventually kill because they have already spread to distant sites in the body before the disease is diagnosed. Local treatments, such as surgery, thus become gates that are closed long after the horse of spreading cancer has bolted.[5]

Had cancer escaped my prostate to reappear in one, five, or ten years?

Clearly, I was to continue to live for years with uncertainty about whether I had been cured or not. And just as clearly, given the accepted lack of knowledge of the causes of my type of cancer, I had to construct my own understanding of why I had gotten cancer, if I were to do anything but submit, to be anything more than a passive observer, even victim, of my life. I have said that I don't submit except on my own terms. So I began a search for possible answers to, "Why me?"

I read Anthony Sattilaro's troubling *Recalled by Life,* and then his *Living Well Naturally.*[6] He had had prostatic cancer that had so spread throughout his system that specialists had given him only a few years to live. He had been castrated and received estrogen therapy. I was not just troubled, but angered. I had found no other book about prostatic cancer and its effects, and he had said nothing about what castration had meant to him and how it had changed his relations with others and his view of himself as a man. He ignored what was just becoming very painful for me—my loss of sexual desire and beginning struggle to live with a dead penis. What captured my interest, though, was his claim to have cured himself by daily yoga and other exercises, meditation, faith, vitamins, and a rigorous macrobiotic diet. Most of his regimens had never been mine. Ten minutes of daily exercise, yes. Earlier efforts to meditate, yes. Now I couldn't even stick to a daily 20 minute meditation period for my talking book. Faith in what? Irish moss? No. And selenium? What was that? His remedies neither appealed to my tastes or schedule nor to my idea of who I was. Even more upsetting was his claim that cancer could be caused by poor diet and a life style whose change required a major reordering of my tastes and priorities. He was for real. No playing around with the cosmetic changes with which I was dallying. He told me, for which I am grateful, that I had to take my way of life much more seriously than I had. I could feel my inner doctor nodding smilingly at that conclusion.

Then I read Charles Simone's book, *Cancer and Nutrition,* a cancer researcher-radiation therapist's critique of available studies of cancer's causes. I had no reason to deny the implications of his prefatory statement, "There is good evidence that 70 to 80 percent of all cancers are produced by diet and nutrition, life-style (smoking, alcohol, etc.), chemicals, and other events in the environment."[7]

So began many hours of thought about why I had gotten cancer and months of effort to reorder my values and ideas about myself.

No family history of cancer. In fact, a genetic history of energetic, healthy parents and grandparents. However, I had not had very emotionally close relations with either of my parents, a familial pattern found in cancer patients but not in other types of patients.[8] I'd had minimal contact with what are now known to be carcinogenic agents: chemicals, tobacco, alcohol, even coffee. My occupation had not yet been identified as causing an increased risk for cancer. And I lived in an environment no more polluted than that of most people who never get cancer. So why me?

I narrowed the probable causes to diet, emotional stress, and my character.

Nutrition? Pete, a close cousin of nutrition faddists and freaks, had suppressed an argument with me for years about one of my few sensuous joys: food, particularly certain foods, which I had eaten with abandon for as long as I could remember. My six-foot frame had never put on excess weight, remaining a constant 170 pounds. And I had eaten without guilt ever since Tom had told me my cholesterol count was so low that I could eat anything! One of my fondest fantasies has always been to make an annual visit to France to dine every night at one of Michelin's three-star gourmet restaurants. I loved heavy cream sauces, homogenized milk, the rich chicken gravies Maryjane made, sausages and gravy for breakfast, fried potatoes, the grease of broiled hamburgers on toasted buns with lots of mayonnaise, brown crinkly skin of broiled chicken, sardine and tuna sandwiches, fresh doughnuts, all forms of eggs, and white bread just out of the oven. I was an old fashioned meat, potatoes, and gravy man. A dinner without meat was not a dinner for me. Broiled marbled steak dripping fat over an open wood fire was really worth living for on a cold winter evening. I was also a dessert person, drawn to any pastry that had sugar and chocolate in it. And I'd eat anything that had real whipped cream on it! A lot of it. And second helpings. I reveled in my high-fat, low-fiber diet.

I definitely was not like Maryjane, who preferred rabbit food: lettuce, salads, barely cooked raw vegetables, apples, yogurt, and sunflower seeds. Or like Pete, who began with brewer's yeast! Yuk.

Sex, nude sunbathing, and my gourmet diet were the only barriers

I had left protecting me from the long hold of my sober Puritan heritage and from emotional death.

Sex was now gone. Sunbathing went several months later as a result of a precancerous skin outbreak. To my dismay, my last sensuous enjoyment was on the verge of dying—all so that I could live?

Moodily defeated, I said to my tape recorder during a bleak moment:

> I enjoy living fully. If I have to live so partially, if my energy is so constrained that I will be constantly preoccupied with myself, if I don't find a deeply fulfilling or satisfying way of living, then I would just as soon not live. Why continue to live, living so dismally? Why leave life on a cheerless note? I want to leave on a long upbeat wave of foaming enjoyment and excitement. I don't want to be a dead living person.

Emotional stress? My type of law was always stressful, for I was ceaselessly involved with the turbulence and pain of people in acrimonious conflict, trying to settle or litigate angry marital disputes or moderate entrenched labor positions. I have lived a high-paced, stressful life for most of the past 20 years. As I became more successful mediating and winning disputes, more intractable and bitter ones only seemed to be attracted to me, particularly in the four years just prior to my cancer. I had been caught in the center of several destructive maelstroms, whirl-pools of viciousness, even attempted murder. My free-wheeling, inno-vative legal efforts drew more clients and more fees than my partners were bringing in. I loved my work, arrived early and stayed late at the office. It was fun, not work. My partners became distant, querulous. And though I was accused by one partner of being a workaholic, I wasn't, for I could surrender my work to play or travel without guilt. Unspoken and ignored, the tension in the firm started interfering with my sleep at night. I began to ask, "Why take this silent treatment to support two of the partners not pulling their weight?" I couldn't resolve the conflict in my own backyard.

Others work in just as intensely provocative jobs. Why should I be the one to get cancer? I'm not sure. But I do have a hunch.

My character? I don't throw off stresses and conflicts. They fes-ter inside, frequently deeply buried, even below my semiconscious mind, only to color my dreams black at night. I've often wished that I were a Harry Truman who reportedly had always been able to sleep at night, even after ordering the bombing of Hiroshima! More telling, I entered too easily into the emotional insides of my clients. I felt what they felt, which meant that every day, in innumerable small ways, I was angry or petulant or despairing or lonely or paralyzed or insulted or hated. I felt some days like the mortician who supposedly dies early because he takes over the mournful blackness of his profession, identifies with it, and slowly wastes away. I was not too well defended against the passions of black and disruptive emotions. The emotional toxins of my daily work had few antidotes. They were seldom expelled, except in those rare moments of courtroom histrionics when I poured my heart out to the jury. But I took its adverse judgments too personally, particularly when I knew without doubt that the verdict was unjust. Where had I failed my client? How could I have argued more persuasively? Once a client committed suicide after the jury went against her. Now I can't even recall her face. That incident had to be left buried wherever it now lies inside.

Reading Lawrence LeShan's *You Can Fight for Your Life* alerted me to my character as a possible contributor to my cancer.[9] He claims that certain types of people get cancer: those who are self-sufficient, independent, unexpressive of their feelings, particularly of hostility and anger. Well, I am like that, but so is almost every man I know. He says those who have experienced a poignant loss are more susceptible. My last major loss was 15 years ago; I mourned it and have never been consciously bothered by it since. So no, that was not me. He cited those who have no long-term purposes or projects and therefore no hope. Definitely not me. I had too many projects to be willing to die yet. He says that those who survive their cancer are the fighters who refuse to accept the verdict that their illness is terminal. Well, I do have a darker, resigned side to my character. I don't know how vigorously I would fight if told I would die in a year or so. I probably would fight, if just to prove the doctors wrong. Yet for weeks I almost succumbed to the foreboding that my cancer would recur and that there was nothing I could do. Maryjane's tearful comment, "That's scary," forced me to consider whether I was not creating just the mental attitude that would fulfill the prediction.

So how did I explain my cancer two months into my healing? Intense persistent interpersonal turmoil, aggravated by my character and not readily shed or diverted away from my body, had over time stressed my immune system. My profligate high-fat, low-fiber diet had brought me too little nourishment. I had had early warnings six years ago that my healing mechanisms were askew when I had prolonged back and abdominal spasms I could not release, only to be followed a year later by 18 months of persistent loose bowel movements I could not cure. And shortly thereafter, in the same lower abdominal area, I had prostatitis and eventually a cancerous prostate. Constitutionally, this area may be where I am most vulnerable to disruptions in my system's functioning. But why cancer of the prostate rather than of the bowel? Poisons can't accumulate there because I am too regular. I half seriously told Maryjane that I had not had enough sex to cleanse my prostate daily!

I now interpret my cancer as a warning that my way of living was becoming so distorted that my body rebelled, saying, "Enough, enough!" Cancer meant a breakdown in my system's healthy integration. I had been living to excess: too much intense emotional conflict not well coped with; too many rich experiences not well digested, needing interpretation and communication; too much identification with the lives of my clients; too busy a schedule; too much focus to listen to my inner voice. I was like that football player who sprains his leg in the first quarter but does not become aware of it until halftime; now it will take much longer to heal than it would have if he had been aware of it earlier. Maybe that is what psychosomatic means: increasing disintegration between our more conscious psychological self and our less conscious but rebelling physical self. This is a verbal distinction I don't really feel in my gut, for the physical was so much the emotional and vice versa for me, I feel uncomfortable talking about the body in opposition to the mind. That's my irrational resistance to dividing myself up into parts, I guess.

Altering my way of life

These emerging attitudes and views about my illness may not meet scientific tests but they told me what I had to do.

My rationality and Puritan will overcame my sensuous self. I began to change my diet and eat like Maryjane and Pete. It took more than a year and a half. Maryjane says that I am not very consistent or faithful to my new diet, but I am remarkably so, given my past habits and character. It is just that I am not a scrupulous ideologue. I am now on a high-fiber and very low-fat diet. And I am enjoying it, though I still hunger for my three-star Michelin gastronomic tour, which I am going to defiantly take when I know I have only a few years left to live. I scarcely eat any of what I used to. I drink skimmed milk, eat only an egg or two a week, and regularly eat bran, rye, and other high-fiber cereals. I have not had sausages and gravy for several years. When I prepare dinner, I think of fruit and vegetable salads, granola muffins, and fish. We have cleaned out the beef and lamb in our freezer. And I occasionally subtitute tofuti for my preferred Breyer's ice cream. I take vitamins A, C, E and selenium every day, though after that first taste the jar of brewer's yeast remains untouched. I was reassured several years after my prostate operation when I found my diet was approaching Sattilaro's ideal for *Living Well Naturally.*

The cancer told me that I had to overthrow the tyranny of my schedule and calendar, reduce emotional stress and conflict, and create a more peaceful work environment. It took months of wrenching thought and small steps to test out my system's reactions, but now in retrospect I see that I was more adaptable than I had thought I could be. So I left my law firm with not one lingering regret, created my own mediation service, accepted clients whose problems would not be so emotionally scarring, and cut out my courtroom appearances.

In addition to continuing my daily exercises, which I have now extended, I joined a health club, where I swim several times a week and work out on the Nautilus equipment. But I still cannot get myself to meditate daily.

I am just as fully engaged in living, but the pacing is radically different, the emotional intensity of my relations with others is less, and my control over my life immeasurably greater. And I am enjoying sunflower seeds!

6
Resilience: The Test of Healing

To mark my progress, I reviewed each month how I was doing. Three months to the day after I lost my prostate, two months after my scheduled recovery, I said:

This dramatic and traumatic spring has now come to a close. Summer is here. Progress? Progress continues slowly, but good days are more frequent than bad ones. I am up, around, active. I'm almost back to my preoperation level of morning exercises. I can now do 40 sit-ups, whereas I couldn't do any three weeks after my operation. I went to the A & P yesterday for the first time wearing underwear, not diapers! Shows some beginning trust in my body and its reliability. The drug I take keeps me dry and already I am beginning to reduce the number of pills I take every day. I have taken over buying food, most of the cooking, and dishwashing. Maryjane is beginning to feel guilty. I am able to work on some of my briefs, but still cannot spend the entire day at the office. I work now more in the evenings, and so am not watching so many movies on the VCR. I can't understand that little lump, though. Sometimes it gets smaller, sometimes larger. It is still painful to sit on. The pain has gradually gone from deep inside to the surface. My scrotum and penis still remain very sore, probably from the drug I am taking to constrict my sphincter muscles. As Tom prescribed, I am vigorously exercising enough to make me breathless; something about expelling poisons? People say I look good. I've begun to test what of my sexuality is left, and am becoming more and more preoccupied by my penis. I feel I am on the verge of a new phase in my healing. I can push my body more and it is more responsive; I feel better about it as I feel more and more alive! Hurrah!

Eight days later hope was demolished. I was right that something new was about to happen, but it wasn't the phase I had expected.

Through the valley of shadows

I sensed something was wrong the moment I saw Dr. Paul. His rectal exam was vigorous as usual, but I didn't wince for the first time since the operation. He was pleased. But he seemed to be preoccupied about something else when answering my usual long list of questions. When I had run out, he ominously began with,

"Mr. Handy. I've been waiting until you were over the infection to tell you that the pathologist had done follow-up studies of your prostate and under other stains found that cancer cells had escaped the prostate."

An eerie numbed feeling swallowed me up. All I could see was his face, which looked sympathetic. Everything else disappeared into blackness.

"We have a scrupulous pathology department. Most other pathologists would never have been so conscientious. He reports cancer cells one millimeter from the edge of the capsule."

What capsule? I had never understood the structure of my prostate, so all I heard was that the cancer had escaped. It was like when he told me I had cancer—I really didn't hear much more. I do recall thinking that one millimeter seemed awfully small. Shit.

"Ten years ago this would never have been picked up. But with new stains and a very compulsive pathology department, well. . . ."

Continued stunned silence.

"I still think you are cured. Because of the operation, there is very limited blood supply to the region, so if cancer did escape it is not likely to survive or grow."

All that I could utter at that moment was, "What do you recommend?"

"Unfortunately, the only study I know of about radiation's effects isn't completed yet and won't be for several years. I've talked with Tom, called other urologists, and consulted with the head of our radiology department. No one knows what to recommend. One consultant said not to tell you, for it would needlessly worry you. The cancer has not metastasized as best as we can tell. It is a micro-metastasis. I still think you are cured."

Feeling weary and defeated, I asked again, almost not caring, "What would you recommend?"

"If it were me, I would get radiation treatment. A low 4000-rad treatment. If you asked other urologists, probably 75 percent of them would say radiation wasn't necessary."

Radiation! To me, emotionally almost as evil as castration. Four-thousand rads, whatever that overwhelming number meant, to my prick and balls, when for years I wouldn't let my dentist give me bite-wings!

My querulous inner doctor prodded me to ask, "How long have you known this?"

"I got the report just before you left the hospital."

"Christ! You've known about this for all of these weeks and never told us? We asked you not to hold anything back from us." Resentfully, I thought of Tom knowing this and not telling me a week before when I had had my annual physical.

"There was nothing you could do. Given your infection, it would have been too risky and too painful to give you radiation. I didn't know if the news might upset your recovery. We had to work on the infection first. Besides, I'm not sure the x-ray therapy department will want to give you cobalt radiation even now."

Trying to suppress my hostility, I asked, "Why not?"

"It can irritate your bowel, possibly cause severe diarrhea, even affect your urination. And you have had surgery there so we don't know how radiation might complicate your continued healing. It could aggravate the pain you've been having."

"Is there anything else you know about me you haven't told me?"

"No."

Dulled and not yet fully understanding what I had been told, I told him I had to talk with Maryjane to decide what to do now.

I dreaded telling her. Fortunately, she had gone to visit her mother and would not be home for two days, giving me time to get more information and settle myself down. When I got home, I told my tape recorder:

I don't know how Maryjane is going to feel. She felt so strongly that we should get the cancer out of my system. I know that affected my judgment. I accept full responsibility for my decision; I do not feel any resentment about her involvement in this whatsoever. I knew what the consequences were and it was the most reasonable decision to make at that time. But in retrospect, we should have had the cobalt treatment. Then I would still have my prostate and be able to have an erection and an orgasm. I probably wouldn't have this leaky penis or have to be on drugs the rest of my life. I did not know that then. I can't regret that decision. But both of us so distrust x-rays and their effects on the body. My system is going to get overloaded with all of this crap. I don't know what to do. I now know some people recover from cancer without all of this treatment. Maybe a change in diet and my way of living would be enough. The real question is, what other systems is the cancer going to invade if it is now loose? More unknowns; more uncertainties. More damned decisions! Goddamn it; here we start all over again.

Maryjane came back a day earlier than planned, apprehensive that something had gone wrong. I sat next to her on the couch with my arm around her as before, and said, "They found cancer in the capsule. No one knows if it has escaped into the lymph." Unbelievable. Tears. Like before.

Then fury: "If they had told us rather than leave us completely in the dark, believing all of this time that they had gotten all of the cancer!" By "protecting" us, Dr. Paul had only set us up for a greater psychological fall. Still crying, she said over and over again, "If only I had had the cancer." The tidal wave had returned. I felt emotionally played out. The early sprigs of hope withered. Not until several weeks later did I understand how much my concentrated focus on my infection and drippy penis had obscured an underlying depression lurking just on the edges of my mind that may have contributed to how strongly I first reacted to the reemergence of such painful uncertainties.

We had been tested once. We had learned from it. So began the same ritual. First, we called Dr. Paul again to clarify what I thought I'd heard. Maryjane was so bitter about our not knowing that I had to step in to divert the discussion. Next, we saw Tom. Yes, prostatic cancer could migrate elsewhere, particularly to the lymph and bones.

Radiation could still be used if cancer had spread outside the prostatic area. We had opted for surgery rather than radiation because we wanted it to be our personal insurance policy in case cancer recurred in the prostatic area. To have had radiation first could have so scarred the prostatic area to make healing from subsequent surgery very doubtful. Our insurance policy had been canceled. If cancer did recur there and radiation was not recommended, then I could be castrated and given estrogen therapy. That joyful prospect. I thought of Sattilaro.

"What would you do?" I asked Tom.

"Have the radiation treatment."

Next, we saw the head of the radiation department, who confirmed what Dr. Paul and Tom had said.

"What are radiation's other effects?"

"Remote possibility of injury to the rectum, possibly to the bladder. Fatigue, diarrhea. And if there were any possibility you could still be potent after the surgery, impotence would be 100 percent certain now."

That last comment chilled me. I had begun to have the warm fantasy that I might be able to stimulate the nerves controlling my erection to regenerate.

"Won't the radiation harm my testicles?"

"No. The machine rotates 360 degrees around you and we can get very precise control of its beam." A drop of relief.

Then I should have another serum acid phosphatase test and another bone scan to see if the cancer had spread in the past three months.

"But why? I just had them. Besides, they are so expensive."

He interpreted the pathologist's report to me. Typical of young men (a characterization the past three months had utterly destroyed), I had had a highly virulent cancer that could spread very rapidly, not the low-grade type that had been clinically diagnosed. I subsequently discovered from reading the urological journals that the severity of prostatic cancer was frequently underestimated clinically, even surgically, when later checked against the pathologist's microscopic findings.[1]

Meanwhile, I was getting very irritable. Maryjane fumed; she was more upset than I have ever seen her. Not trusting Dr. Paul now, my advocate sought out other professional opinions. Yes, he had an excellent reputation among other urologists, which was comforting. She then insisted we get a second opinion. I didn't think it necessary, but my intuitive physician told me that she needed reassurance.

The next evening, I asked the consultant, somewhat puzzledly, "If Dr. Paul thinks I am cured, then why is he recommending I get radiation?"

"He may feel sure from what he observed during the operation but intuitively he may feel he didn't get all of the capsule out. Besides, he may be just very conservative and not want to take any chances." Sounded reasonable to me.

"Are there any dangerous effects of radiation?"

"Maybe a five-percent chance of permanent damage to the urethra or lower bowel."

Damn. So many uncertainties.

"How effective will radiation be now?"

"We don't know. Might improve your chances of not having a recurrence of cancer by five to ten percent."

I had to keep in mind this was a urologist speaking. I already knew that there were disputes between radiologists and urologists about the effectiveness of their different treatments.

"What is the recurrence rate of this type of cancer?"

"Within five years, about two-thirds of the patients will still be living."

A cold shudder went through me. I felt Maryjane wince. Blunt, direct, straightforward—what we wanted. But it hurt. At least this figure was better than the fifty-percent chance I had earlier read about.

"What can I do to prevent recurrence?"

"Nothing."

Another blow. I took in a deep breath. To tell me there is nothing I can do is like waving a red flag in front of a bull. Even though I may now be an impotent bull, I am not one to submit and do nothing. Dr. Paul and Tom later also said, "Nothing." I felt that something close to the core of my being was being tested. Was faith all that was left?

"What about potency? Anything I can do to try to regenerate the nerves?"

"No. Radiation will take away whatever small chance you now have of regaining your potency."

Walking out into the warm summer evening, I shivered. My hands were cold. I reached out to take Maryjane's always-warmer hand. Hers was cold too. Silently, we walked to the car cold hand in cold hand.

What was to happen?

What were we to decide? We had been through this valley before. More uncertainties. I tersely summarized them this way to my recorder that evening:

> Now I may have or may not have cancer cells in my body. If I do, the cells may or may not be viable. If viable, they may grow only in the prostatic area or they may migrate. If they grow they may not become a clinical problem for years. If they migrate, they could go to my bones, my brain. They may already have migrated. Radiation to the prostatic area may finally kill those damn killers; it might miss them if they have already migrated. I may not know for years, if ever (then I don't care!), where I may next get signs of cancer. The radiation may, though improbably, create permanent damage to my bowel and urethra. It could shrink my bladder, which is already incapable of holding more than half a cup of urine. All hope of regaining my erection will be gone.

The same bottom-line question decided for us. If I did not get the five-week, 4000-rad treatment the radiologist planned, and if cancer recurred, how could we live together realizing the treatment might have prevented its recurrence? The wisdom of our decision to get the radiation was confirmed several years later. During a bi-monthly trek through the recent urological journals I discovered studies claiming that when the capsule had been penetrated, radiation therapy could produce very favorable results, particularly if initiated within four months of surgery.[2]

Again, we called Lucy and Pete. Disbelief. Anger. Others we called reacted as they had when they first heard of my cancer, only this time with less intensity, as if this might be routine.

I felt resigned, even accepting.

I began the measurements for the computer determinations of the coordinates and daily dosage the next day. Two days later, treatments started. Five days a week for five weeks, I drove to the hospital, took off my pants and underwear, got into another one of those skimpy gowns, went to the john, sat down to wait for my turn, entered the windowless room where I climbed awkwardly to lie flat on my back on a table under the x-ray machine. Not one of those 25 days was

I free from worrying that the radiologists might slip up in their coordinate settings and direct those silent, deadly, though painless, rays onto my defenseless penis and testicles. At least I didn't have to fret about what my penis would do when the young nurses uncovered me down there and occasionally brushed the covering against it. It behaved impeccably, no thanks to my desire or will. It was tested daily. Regretfully—no, sorrowfully—it passed every test. It would never again be disobedient!

During those hot, humid, interminable five weeks, I saw myself slowly retreating from the good feeling I had had about myself just before I entered the valley of shadows. The radiologist was right. My stamina started to go about the third week. My genital area became annoyingly sensitive and painful. Diarrhea required me to go off the fruits and vegetables I had begun to like and resume eating white bread and other foods less abrasive to my bowel. I retreated back along the route my healing had taken up to this point. I turned back into myself and spent more time talking to my recorder. More vulnerable emotionally, I did not want to talk with others for any length of time, saw my partners less frequently, puttered around the house when I had the energy, took more frequent naps, went to bed earlier. And waited.

Maryjane drove me to my last treatment. High expectations. Excitement. Finally, freedom from the hospital, doctors, radiation. We were going to leave for our summer place, where I expected my real healing to begin. I would really be on my own. But luck fled again. The hospital did not want to lose its grip on me. A fuse blew, not to be replaced for 75 minutes, while a fuming, impatient Rich Handy did not have the decency, or resources, to hide his irritability from the hapless nurses. I failed this test flat out. Then, washed out, aching in my lower abdomen as a result of the accumulated radiation, I lay for six hours in the back of the car, unable to help Maryjane with the driving. I had to stop at every gas station along the turnpike, for I had vowed never to wear those diapers again!

Resiliency to testing

The recurrence of the shadowy unknowns that I had put aside and even cleared away tested my emotional stability, my resiliency. In three months I had traveled from acute vulnerability through numerous, frequently unpredictable, dark and dismal moods, to more sunny, even joyful moments. During one depressing period along the way, five weeks after entering the hospital, I said:

My mood is low. I am close to tears. I feel them, though they never come. Today, stormy, occasionally sharp claps of thunder outside. Spring seems to be coming so slowly this year. Just a thin green. The daffodils are just coming out. Some tulips are on the way. But we have not had a really warm sunny spring day since I have come home. I guess my mood is influenced by that. Like spring's, my progress is really so slow. Maryjane says I have to think in terms of months, not weeks. She is right, of course. I have to keep in perspective what has happened to me.

Five days later:

Celebration. For the second time I have been dry most of the night. I am wearing the same diaper all morning. It is now two o'clock in the afternoon and I am only slightly wet, which means my involuntary muscle is beginning to function. There is hope ahead.

I never became so paralyzed by despair that I could not function; nor did I ever give up or lose hope. Perhaps because I could not really believe the reality of what I was experiencing, I still had not "owned" the cancer in me. I bounced back similarly to the shock of the pathologist's gloomy news.

Three days after I began cobalt radiation:

I am somewhat stoical now. I am pleased that I will be able to continue working, though at a reduced level of efficiency. I do not have to cancel all of my court appearances and stop work on my other cases. I slept well last night, so maybe I have accepted my new fate. I am not fighting it. I have not stayed angry or been plunged into a more severe depression.

Months later when typing this reaction from the tape, I noted:

I find typing this is plummeting me into a very low, sad mood. But I am puzzled why on the tape I talked so briskly, objectively, matter-of-factly, with no anger or depression in my voice, so sharp, even aggressive, but very detached. Where were my feelings about this devastating news?

This comment captured both a strength and a weakness in my character. I knew that I bounced back quickly from shocks; I could rely on that to get me through the next weeks. I would cope. I also knew that I was in a different emotional place now than I had been at the time of my operations. They had put me through much worse than what radiation promised; it would be silent and painless, and its visible results would likely not be as dramatically crippling as the surgery's incontinence and impotency. At worst, the radiation would only confirm both.

For three months, I had slowly begun to regain trust in my body. It had become more dependable; more energy had become freed to cope with other issues. I had become much less frequently emotionally upset, even when talking with Pete. I had felt my "old" energetic, lively, affectionate self returning. If I put the two neatly stitched cloth-covered stacks of *National Geographic*s that Maryjane had made under my spread legs, I could drive the car again. I couldn't control my urine without a drug but at least I knew I could manage to appear in court again. I was regaining trust in my body, enough even to drive to the A & P without wearing a diaper! So trivial, yet so reassuring. That trust in the predictability of my body, in my emotional reactions, gave me confidence to risk traveling further and further, though for months I still took diapers along with me just in case. The injury to my self-trust had penetrated so deeply that even now, five years later, I still keep four unused diapers in my closet—just in case!

Bouncing back so quickly could be a weakness, however, as my inner physician knew. It could get in the way of the deeper healing I intuitively sensed I had yet to go through if I were to become more whole. I had to give up what had been cancer-inducing in my life, mourning not only those losses, but also the death of my penis, and maybe the end of my life as well.

Trust to mourn

Perhaps because of being so turned inward, so focused on mv physical recovery, so worried about the infection, and so preoccupied about my incontinence, I had had no energy left to mourn. Up and down moods, yes. But no mourning. For three pre-radiation months my intuitive guide had known that I was not yet strong enough to face the losses I had had and would have in the future. Just prior to being informed about the cancer's escape, I had felt that I was in much stronger shape than before. I had reached a more stable level of physical wholeness. I had felt my stability and resiliency returning and so was more hopeful about the future—despite the gloomy statistics about survival rates. I was now strong enough to follow the mourning trail of the three revelations and paradoxically to risk "falling apart" emotionally along the way.

Dr. Paul's announcement upset my inner physician's emotional timetable. He insisted once again that I postpone exploring the meaning of my impotence until I approached the end of my radiation treatments.

"Dick, don't explore those three revelations yet. Slow down and keep working on controlling your urine. The radiation is likely to set you way back in that task if you don't keep persisting. Leave the loss of your erection until later. The radiation will sap your ability to withstand the pain in those memories."

I consciously refused to let Old Faithful's death into my mind those early weeks. It was the right decision to have made, though hints of what I was to face kept occasionally trespassing into my awareness as the radiation continued.

Outwardly, I kept going. As I neared the end of radiation, continuously struggling to control my urine, I inwardly and hesitantly began to mourn: four months for Old Faithful's death, five months beyond that for my own, though initially only fragmentarily. While only Maryjane knew, sensitive Lucy perceived my inner struggle; she visited very frequently, asking what was wrong. I couldn't tell her. I barely knew myself. I let myself be drawn into this depressive period because I felt I could finally trust myself to go where I had to go—into the meaning of the three revelations about what my former cock had meant to me, and only after that, into the meaning of my own dying.

Part III
Meditations on Maleness

I still feel awe about what are, to me, two miraculous facets of my inner physician's skill in directing my healing. Over and over I sensed whether or not it was time to take a given step. His timing seemed to be impeccable. And over and over I marveled at how I seemed to be repeating a journey I had taken before. Not just in how my healing proceeded for each phase, but also in how each phase seemed to follow naturally from the preceding one. For example, the operations had made me a helpless baby, vulnerable to and very dependent upon an intrusive world. My consciousness lost its dimensionality and so its perspective. And though my sense of self temporarily dissolved, I quickly began to develop barriers to protect its fragility.

Like an infant who must trust others in order to grow, I turned, in the presence of healing others, to connect with the world around me. As I began to assert my will, test what my body could and could not do, and learned to control my urination and defecation again, I regained trust in its reliability. It no longer embarrassed me, caused me doubt, or absorbed so much energy to monitor. Trust in my body's basic survival capacities freed me to begin to discover what the death of Old Faithful meant to me as a male and how I was to relate to others. This path was a long and rocky one, and it was over a year after my radiation before I completed it.

My inner physician's three revelations remarkably charted the course my healing next took, reliving first the childhood, then the adolescent, and finally the adult meanings of my formerly very alive cock, now a very dead penis. The first revelation took me back to my pre-pubertal self when I had discovered the pleasures of my emergent sexuality. The second plunged me into very troubling emotional recesses and the unfinished adolescent tasks of experimenting with how to connect with other males. Only after reliving this period was I ready to understand the third revelation, my relationships with females, and to answer the question, "How am I to love Maryjane now?"

7
The First Revelation:
Discovery of Sexuality

I was nine years old, lying on my back in a tub of warm water taking my evening bath. Suddenly, with no warning and for no reason, my penis started to get bigger, harder. It raised itself up to snuggle against my stomach. This had never happened before. I was amazed, awed, scared! What was wrong? I had lived with this penis and taken it for granted for nine years. What was it doing, acting like that? It wouldn't go down. I squeezed it to make it go down; it only got harder. How could I walk around with this hard thing sticking out? I became embarrassed. What would others think if they saw it? I didn't feel panicky; it just made me feel too good, warm, the way I felt when I teased a girl at school whom I thought I loved. I just lay there, watching, puzzled. My hard penis felt so good I just knew it couldn't be bad; it became my secret delightful mystery. I didn't even know words for what I was feeling: "penis," "erection," even "sex" had never been used in my family home and never would be. This left a lot of room for a vivid imagination and unselfconscious exploration later on in my teens.

It was not until I precipitiously lost my erection that I understood how central my cock had been to my identity as a male. How silently it had inched its way into most nooks and crannies of my view of myself, as the themes of my first revelation were to show me 43 years later. What had I been before the operation?

Before

When I was younger, my soft but plump 4½ inches excited respect from others, such as the young man I had never seen before, who said after seeing me shower after a workout in the college pool, "You have a lot of muscle there." It was a penis others would look at in locker rooms. I was proud of it and did not try to hide my treasure from myself or from others. I was well hung, in today's language. Because my penis was so warmly full, I enjoyed holding it. I used it as my portable handwarmer during cold winter nights.

When hard, my penis stretched itself into about 6½ inches from its tip to my pubic bone. When I was younger, it held its head very high; as I grew older, it remained sturdy and firm, though its angle of inclination became less, about 80 degrees before my operation. It did curve, though, slightly to the left.

Old Faithful had seldom let me down; only a few times the year before the operation. I did not know how fortunate I had been until I read the Hite report, one of the few intensive (though possibly flawed) surveys yet done of male sexual attitudes and beliefs, which had appeared a year earlier.[1] Apparently 64 percent of the participating males reported difficulty in having erections when they wanted them. Like the cocks of many men, mine responded both when I wanted it to and when I didn't. Easily arousable, it was responsive to the most trivial, puzzling, and embarrassing situations. I got a hard-on the first time I smoked a cigarette. Maryjane's slightest touch could make it fly. I often marveled at her control over my "love." Even while visiting a French beach, I had to spend most of my time lying on my stomach. My bikini provided little camouflage. I ached for hours afterward. Visiting the Greek sections of museums was always an unpredictable sexy adventure. My cock's psychopathic lack of discrimination, even guilt, remained a constant torment to my conscience during my adolescent and early adult years.

My eager cock caused me much embarrassment when I was young. (If only it had had the same potential for mischief in my later years!) One day in math class when I was 14, it unpredictably raised its head when I was called upon to work a problem on the blackboard. To this day, I shy away from writing on blackboards in front of others. Taking showers after gym class too frequently became a test of my budding willpower, which just as frequently I failed. I still blush recalling that night I was showering in my dorm's bathroom. Without any help or thought from me, I spontaneously got a magnificent hard-on. (Due, my revelation tells me, to being nude in warm water, which has always made me feel sensuous.) Some guys from down the hall who were horsing around outside suddenly burst into the shower room. I hastily turned my back, cursing indiscreet Old Faithful. They insisted on staying there for an interminable time, talking about what I don't recall; I tried to answer, turning my head but shielding my betrayer. They were kinder than some other friends would have been; they knew I was vulnerable.

What shame my cock has brought me. I retreated from team sports in the seventh grade, due in part to my apprehension about what it was going to do next. I became so tensely modest that I dreaded undressing in front of others. As I grew older and its eagerness became less insistent, I learned to enjoy hot steam baths, stretching out stark naked, which reaffirmed my sensuous maleness. Any new adventure could provoke Old Faithful to remind me of his presence—like the first time I leaned forward to kiss a girl and missed her mouth because I was simultaneously preoccupied with how to prevent Old Faithful from meeting her.

My cock had a more functional use, though I regret I was so old in discovering it. When I was 16 and showering after a swim with a friend, he reached out to touch Old Faithful and teach it how to spout. My reaction? Dumbfounded amazement. Extraordinary. "This is great!" I subsequently learned that my nervous system is very easily excited. I called it "my autonomic instability." I discovered that Old Faithful could provide a marvelously pleasurable and free tranquilizer for my "on edge" nervous system. I learned to use it frequently, particularly during times of great stress, like before taking exams at college or when anticipating a difficult court case. Old Faithful's spouting calmed me down. From my early thirties on, my body has needed at least two relaxation treatments a week—even more when I am in new, exciting settings, like with Maryjane on our "honeymoon" vacations.

How does a man live with such a willful, responsive cock? Not until it died, paradoxically in the service of keeping me alive a little while longer, did I appreciate what it had done to and for me. And how much energy I had spent in learning to live with it.

After

What was I like after my operation? For months, my soft penis remained a shriveled, one-inch, infant-like replica of the penises on statues of cherubs. I so despaired at how deeply hidden my pride had become amid its foreskin that I sought medical advice. I could not even put two fingers around it. It had become ugly, purplish, wrinkled, and dribbly. I winced when I saw it in the mirror. It reminded me that I'd had cancer, so I avoided looking at it for weeks.

It permanently lost its cockiness. It died and became only a limp penis. I no longer felt any sexy pleasure in it, only painful soreness. Whereas before my cock had been a lively, unpredictable source of emotion, now it was like a small lifeless toe. I could wiggle every other part of my body except it and my ears. I could no longer daydream some sexual adventure and make it tingle and stretch. It just passively drooped. I became very "safe" around others.

So what secrets did I discover about the meanings of my former erections and my maleness?

Erections equal excitement and aliveness: "I was amazed, awed, scared!"

For six weeks after the operation, I existed, feeling about 35 percent alive, 65 percent sore, pained, washed out. I couldn't even enjoy physically stretching my muscles; I could scarcely do several sit-ups. I did not feel good, warm, excited. I did not feel sexy at all, would have no desire to have sex with Maryjane for months, and so thought that impotence had destroyed my sexual desire and responsiveness. Another fruit of my ignorance! So one afternoon while lying in bed, I experimented by drawing my fingers gently over my nipples, chest, and arms. And for the first time felt warm, good, even a tingle. Excitedly, I caressed my penis. I felt nothing. Dead. Confirmation of despair!

I later reflected about this:

I now realize that "erotic" had been too narrowly focused a word for me. It really means that good, healthy, vibrant feeling when the body is working well, when stroking the skin makes one feel excited, alive, moved. I wonder if I have to feel good, sensuous pleasure in my body *before* I can be aroused sexually. I don't think erotic feelings can be separated from feeling good about being alive. They certainly don't mean only having a sexy erection.

My memory of my first erection, my reaction to warm showers, even waking with a hard-on in the morning, told me that my erections meant I was aroused, excited, alive, not just sexually desirous.

Perhaps because the cancer and its treatment involved my more erotically sensitive parts—my penis and anal area, even my bladder and rectum—I became oversensitive to their changing erotic messages. The muted pleasurable sensual sensations my healing body slowly returned to me made me feel more and more alive. Putting on a diaper gave me a tinge of the same excited feeling that putting on a jock strap had always given me. Squatting to be able to get my two wayward urinary streams into the toilet made me feel sensuous. Some of my daily exercises sensitized me to deeply erotic feelings and memories, even programmed reflexive patterns underlying my former orgasms. To strengthen my abdominal muscles, I put my hands behind my head, thrust out my pelvis, and tightened my buttocks, making me very aware of sensuous and increasingly sexy sensations in this area. I began to monitor my return to life by how my sensuousness became increasingly more focused sexually. I will always remember the moment when bracing my hands against the sides of the door jamb, holding my shoulders back, and thrusting my pelvis through the door, I thought of entering Maryjane. The first hard sign of sexual desire's return.

Nine months of vulnerability and self-conscious awareness of my body's travail and its inner movement led to these comments about my eroticism:

I had a sexy dream last night and woke up holding my penis. Lying in bed this morning I thought of my erotic feelings. They are the ground of my being, emerging when I am relaxed or sleeping, when I am away from the hold my work has on me, when traveling and tired, when I see an attractive person. It is as if I am primed at a low level to become aroused and diffusely excited. My eroticism is the background "noise," the unspoken dynamic, the underground stream of life. Since so much of my life is concentratedly focused on projects, brief after brief, arguments, connecting to others and to the world around me, I am not usually aware of this underground stream. My life's dominant figure is adapting, coping, achieving, externalizing preoccupations. Only at those moments when the figure slips away, like during these past months, does the underground erotic stream flow into consciousness. I don't consciously think of myself as a sexy, sensuous, earthy, passionate person, though sometimes after a court trial, some tell me they felt I had been carried away by too much excitement—the conversion of the erotic into forceful impetuous intellectual energy, the flowing and channeling of the hidden stream into more focused activity.

When I typed out my talking book, I noted that in the first month of my recovery, the erotic, the feeling of excited aliveness, was completely absent. Only a few references had been made to impotence. Then a few spasmodic references to sexual feelings. After about five weeks I began to say I was feeling good for the first time, that I was less absorbed by my body. And about this time I began to explore my sexuality. Every time I was depressed or in pain the erotic took flight.

I have always intuitively felt that there was a connection between this underground erotic stream and creativity. When I am turned deeply inward, unaware of the claims of the world around me, relaxed, meditative, I can be flooded with ideas as I feel the eroticism of my nature bubbling up into awareness.

I had always felt most alive when I had erections, even when I awoke in the morning with no thought of sex in mind. They brought spice, vitality, adventure to living. My illness and impotence reminded me of that. Erections had told me that life has its ups and downs. They created inner tumult and excitement, disturbed me, forced me to leave home, to get away from being only with myself. My erections provoked me to become an intruder. They got me into all kinds of adventures. When I was young, they drove me to restlessly explore, to walk the streets, to try to connect with others, more often than not, not knowing what I was seeking. My erections demanded I do something about their claims, not just for release but also for connecting with others. They made me emotional, excited, restless. They demanded new growth.

For many younger males, erections mean not just aliveness but life itself, the life they and their semen can bring to women. Thankfully, I never had to face the emotionally devastating possibility of not being able to produce a child. Erection as a symbol of fertility was no longer part of my psyche. The phase of wanting to produce children was now well behind me, so I did not have to mourn that loss.

Erections equal sexual desire: "The way I felt when I teased a girl at school whom I thought I loved."

Profusely sprinkled among my seven months of meditations are many laments about not feeling any strong sexual desire or impetus to seek out sexual relations. Seventy days after my operation, I morosely said to myself, "Rationally, I have had to admit that the prospects are less and less that I will ever again have much sexual pleasure." Yet, on the 27th postoperative day my returning eroticism was focusing more and more on sex. That day, I said:

> In the bath this morning, I felt my penis getting fuller and had the fantasy that I was going to have an erection. My penis does vary in size, so there is blood flowing to it. It is just that the erectile reflex is missing. I feel it getting hard but am surprised when I look and find it isn't.

By the fifth week, while taking my first postoperative shower, I had the urge to masturbate, which I attempted several times a week from then on, without any noticeable effect. I began to get some sexy feelings from exercising, started to make sexy jokes with Maryjane, and had transparently sexual dreams.

It took me 14 weeks to figure out this paradox; I had no strong sexual desire and yet was acting sexy. Like many men, I had identified how sexually desirous I was with how hard my cock was. To me, no erection meant no sexual desire! It had taken me years to associate "desire" with erections. Erections at nine years of age while bathing in the tub or at 11 and 12 while having a free-for-all gang wrestle were exciting, enjoyable, and, thankfully, shameless reactions to have, but they did not drive or motivate me to seek such excitement. By 16, when I learned how great an ejaculation was, I began to "desire" and seek more. Though I'd had an erection in the college shower without any conscious desire, I knew by this time that it was being interpreted, by those who saw it and by me, as sexual arousal.

I also figured out that feeling or seeing my penis hard was a powerful cue that initiated and heightened my sexual desire and alerted me to my body's attraction to someone. Much as I loved dancing when I was young, I was always apprehensive that my date might rub up against me too closely. During adolescence I also became excited by observing other males' erections, even dogs', horses', and bulls'. Becoming firm was a very reliable cue to my sexual desire, and seeing and touching my cock only excited my desire even more.

My impotence disrupted this complex physio-emotional pattern. I now did not have my most reliable clue about how I was feeling, nor did I receive any intense stimulation of desire from my limp penis. I also learned that when my penis did grow bigger, as it did when I was relaxing in the bathtub or before going to sleep at night, from a shy one-inch recluse to a brazen 4½-inch snake creeping down to the bottom of my scrotum, I began to feel more sexy. This sexiness, though, made me increasingly wistful, even sad, since my expectant hopes that my penis would suddenly rear up were never fulfilled.

Worried about my lagging sexual desire, I read a book recommended by Dr. Paul, Sherman Silber's *The Male*.[2] He claimed that though the male hormone secreted by the testicles contributes to sexual desire, increases in the hormone do not lead to increased desire. Also, erectile potency is independent of testosterone level. Erections can occur without accompanying sexual desire and vice versa, as I had discovered. I now attribute my muted and delayed sexual desire not to damage to the testicles from the radiation I had so feared, but primarily to the absorption of my energy by the healing process, which left little strength for sexual expression. And what squanders sexual energy as quickly as an orgasm? My sexual desire returned in full force only with increased physical and mental healing, especially after I emerged out of a prolonged depression.

Erections equal orgasms: "It just made me feel too good, warm."

For months I suffered from ignorance about my body. Since it had always worked reliably, I'd never had to know much about it. Intellectually I knew that though I would never ejaculate again, I *could* have an orgasm. Emotionally I did not know that. I knew nothing about the mechanism of an orgasm. Like the 66 percent of men in Hite's report, I confused erection, ejaculation, and orgasm. Hite claimed that only 16 percent of those who answered her questionnaire knew that a man could have an orgasm without an ejaculation. Old Faithful had *always* erupted until about a year prior to my cancer, when often I could no longer feel myself ejaculating during lovemaking.

My confusion was only confirmed when I stroked my shrunken penis for the first time, five weeks after my operation:

> I feel really quite low and pessimistic. I dug myself into this mood because I became increasingly curious, for I am going to have to deal very soon with my impotence. To learn if I can have an orgasm, I took a shower and tried to masturbate. Nothing happened, even when I used an oil that used to stimulate me. I did not even feel aroused, let alone sexy. I feel devastated. I'll continue to test my body. Who knows, maybe I'll be able to regenerate some nerves or some miracle will occur and bring back the feelings that have meant so much to me in the past. I feel like I am in puberty again trying to figure out what my body is and is not, what it can and cannot do.

Nothing had changed twelve days later when I asked Dr. Paul what had happened to my orgasms. He assured me they would come back. Big sigh and a grin. But I asked myself, "How in the hell do I have one since I no longer can get an erection and ejaculate?"

I kept persisting, doing all kinds of things to my penis and experiencing only occasional twinges of pleasure. A few days after beginning radiation, I tried once again and nothing happened. I said:

> It left me irritable and tense. I had no reaction whatsoever. I must be very careful not to try to stimulate my body when it is not ready to respond. It is a great temptation to do so because I want to find out. Will I ever feel an orgasm again? What is happening to this core of my vitality? Am I too impatient, as Maryjane keeps insisting? The odds now do not seem to be favorable that my body is going to be very responsive in the future. Dr. Paul and the consultant said I should have recovered a long time ago. I try to act as if my body will be responsive and it isn't. Just another one of those small nails

being driven into my coffin of despair. I had better relax with my body, stop driving it to do something it may not be ready to do.

But I couldn't relax. The next week I began to get uncontrollable muscle twitches in my legs and arms while going to sleep or during the night. My entire body became spasmodic, almost as I were going into a seizure. Was my weary, frustrated body telling me that it too wanted to have an orgasm, to discharge a lot of accumulated tension? I couldn't help it out. Intensive physical exercise helped, but my jerking and twitching continued to disturb my sleep for weeks.

And then it happened! After a particularly severe spell of spasms one night, I tried to tranquilize my body once more. Suddenly I shouted to Maryjane. "I'm having an orgasm! I'm having an orgasm!" I didn't even mind that it was so muted, that I didn't know when I had "come," since I had no ejaculation. I only really knew when I continued to masturbate and became very irritable. Then I relaxed emotionally. I had arrived. I had crossed another threshold; it was like the first time I'd had sexual intercourse. I finally knew that my basic neurological programming was still intact. I had my tranquilizer back, though it surely wasn't an earthshakingly pleasurable experience taking it!

When I know that my car isn't quite right, I become hyper-alert to its every sound. So I became ultra-sensitive to every small "noise" my returning orgasmic capability made. Its slow restoration took months, though extraordinary and sometimes violently intense stimulation was required to get it to speak to me above a whisper. I had never before masturbated anything but an engagingly responsive, stoutly firm cock. Now I had to learn what to do with a meager one-to-four-inch, apathetic, utterly limp penis. It makes me blush to report how exhaustively I explored my past imaginative masturbatory history for four "adolescent" months to find the keys that might unlock that orgasm and free it to take climactic possession of me. I suppose that by this time psychiatrists could have told me where to search, but I had to follow the path that my inner doctor was revealing.

What is an orgasm like to an impotent man at this stage in his recovery? One hundred and thirty-five days after I lost my erection, I finally decided that I could have an orgasm, as subdued as it was. I described it this way:

Every three or four days I become restless and irritable. I begin to think, "Maybe I should try masturbating again to see if any of these feelings are coming back, to see if the experience of orgasm is different." My sexual desire is not focused toward people, only toward my body. I don't trust my body in a relationship with another yet. I would find such efforts to be irritating and probably painful, possibly shattering my fragile feelings about myself. My erotic energy is not yet freed from my preoccupation with my body to be able to give it to another.

My "orgasms" are getting easier to have. Just as I am about to have a very quiet ripple of a climax my abdomen tenses, I instinctively thrust and thrust, my body begins to stiffen but not with the self-abandonment I was used to, nothing like the totally physical kind of giving, responding, and dimming of consciousness that I remember. It is very focused, an abbreviated analogue. I feel no great rush, no intense pleasure. Maybe Masters and Johnson [whom I had read to find out what I should have been feeling] were right when they said that intensity of sexual pleasure is caused by the amount of semen being ejaculated. I have only dry runs now, followed by a deep lassitude, the only word I can use to describe the result.

So the basic components are there: heightening of tension, pelvic thrusting, bodily stiffening, painful irritability if I continue too long, and lassitude. Now instead of ejaculation, irritability is to be forever the substitute sign that I have had an orgasm. Great!

My problem is, how in the hell do I transfer this feeling, as mild as it is, into a relationship with someone else when I can't have a hard-on? I've talked about this with Maryjane, who suggests I see a sex therapist. I'm not interested. I need to understand more the limits of my body, what it is capable and not capable of, and reestablish enough trust to be able to submit with abandonment to my body's demands. I feel I have to go through that whole adolescent self-discovery ritual, but focused now on a particular part of me that is no longer me. This whole episode has shaken my confidence in who I am and what I can do with my body; it has created such uncertainty that I can't trust myself. I still do not know with certainty that I can get to the john in time without making a mess—which happened again yesterday.

Erections equal wary control: "It wouldn't go down. I squeezed it to make it go down. . . . I became embarrassed."

My willful, unpredictable cock had become a symbol of my autonomic instability and intense emotionality. Inwardly, I react strongly and quickly. I reach out to touch others too soon when I meet them. Tears come too easily. Troubles with a client often bother me so that I can't sleep. Irritability and anger well up quickly. The operations stirred up my inner vulnerabilities, which showed in my reactions to Pete and others. I became easily irritated and impatient: when I couldn't pass an elderly woman poking along below the speed limit; with the recorded telephone message, "Please wait. All of our reservation agents are busy"; with clients who wandered in tedious circumstantial detail and wouldn't get to the point; with the telephone company repair man who insisted that he could not get my telephone fixed until the following week. I fumed. After one of these episodes, the doctor recorded my blood pressure at 145 over 90, when it normally rested around 115 over 80. I wondered if the recurring thought, "I don't have much time left," was making me more emotional.

I never so condemned my emotional responsiveness and cocky waywardness to push them out of consciousness, like many American males do. As the first revelation showed, I treasured my "secret delightful mystery," my emotional sexy self. I still do. But I had to make it "secret," by learning such self-control that I could appear to be what I was not. So began years of creating all kinds of inner complications by which to live in a society that did not allow its males emotionality, affectionate demonstrativeness, tears, or alive, wandering cocks.

The outcome of years of learning how to consciously delay, suppress, control, discipline my cock was the development of a strong will. Like my former cock, I had become "will-full." I meditated at length on why I so struggled with the issue of control throughout my healing:

Much of my will has come from trying to master my cock. When I was 16, 17, 18, and 19, the temptations to masturbate were so intense that I had to struggle to resist, with much guilt over my failure to control my own body. One day, I just gave up, saying, "What's wrong with feeling good? If that is what my body wants, then it needs it."

I feel that there is some relationship between my will and my control of this unpredictable part of my body. It led to a hyper-modesty about my sexuality in relation to both males and females, because I couldn't trust what my reactions might be. I don't know how, but this drive to control my erections seems to have become intertwined with a whole complicated network of feelings and reactions to other people. I wonder if the unpredictability and uncontrollability of erections make men more sexually centered than women. I am certainly more sexually preoccupied than Maryjane is. She doesn't have to worry about unpredictably revealing to others her sexual desire. I facetiously told her that I thought God made me, as a male, stand upright so she could tell just how much of a male I was and when I was lusting after her.

Impotence meant my penis was now so reliable that it was no longer mischievous. It had become boring. Although it used to be temperamental and unruly, I'd still had some control over it. I had learned how to make it hard or soft. Now I couldn't. What did this mean to me?

With a tone of nostalgic sadness, even hints of defiance, I fruitlessly repeated near the end of my radiation treatments another one of my experiments to test my control of Old Faithful:

> I have lost control of the variable part of me. It has become a constant, no longer unpredictable. Something that is always constant is without emotion; constancy washes out feelings. I feel much less emotionally sensitive now. My erotic reactions are so muted that I no longer have the same desire to connect with others. In the past I could make my penis raise its head by imagination alone. Damn it!' I'll make it do that now. [Pause followed by an expression of sad resignation.] I can't even get blood down there at all. It doesn't quiver. What shall I do? What could I think of doing to make it get bigger? [Pause] I can't do anything. It just lies there. I have lost control of a central part of me. All it is now is a conduit for urine; for sex it is nothing. Nothing happens. I have become powerless. An impotent male who has lost the core of his excitement and vitality. What meaning is left?

Erections equal male pride: "How could I walk around with this hard thing sticking out?"

Of course, my three revelations show that I *wanted* to walk around with my "hard thing sticking out," since it is the symbol of my maleness. In the first revelation, I was obviously fascinated by my cock snuggling up near my belly button; in the second, secretly pleased though outwardly conflicted about having my cock chosen for the group demonstration of adult maleness; and in the third, proud enough to tie a red bow on it as my Christmas present to Maryjane—giving my love to her!

Like having one's breast, hand, or leg amputated or becoming very disfigured, losing the ability to have erections must alter a normal male's view of himself. To what extent such a shock traumatizes depends, of course, upon how important the lost or maimed body part was to the person. Maybe my formerly sexy and tranquilizing cock had been more important to me than most other men's are to them. I don't know. The men I know never talk about such personal things. When they do, they speak in such a macho, crude, joking way, I don't know how to read how they really feel. And I personally don't know any impotent males willing to talk about what the loss of their erection has meant to them. Even the medical profession seems tongue-tied about the issue; at least, none of my doctors could tell me anything useful.

As I said, not until my cock had died did I realize how central it had been to my identity. I unconsciously but much too often began to refer to myself as "crippled." For months I drove to the local A & P and thought I had a right to park in the spot marked "handicapped." I resisted the temptation when I thought about trying to explain to a policeman why I had parked there. I had not realized how firmly anchored my unconscious image of my maleness had been to my erection. Maryjane said there was much more to living than the ability to have an erection. Rationally, I replied, "Of course," but I didn't believe her.

The Hite report reassured me, however, that many other males felt about their cocks as I did about mine. I now understand in my gut why an opening scene in the movie, *Yankee,* brought me close to tears. In it a young soldier who'd had both legs amputated wrote euphemistically to his girlfriend back home, "But the most important thing was saved." I understand why one man told me that he *had* to get a penile implant because he "felt like only half a man." And why some men report that after they lose their erections they feel that they have died. In his book, *Male Sexual Function*, Dr. Richard Milsten, a urologist, poignantly illustrates what some impotent men feel:

"I don't feel like a complete man."

"I always wondered what it would be like to be without a penis. Now I know. It's there but it only hangs and doesn't seem to be useful for any purpose except going to the bathroom. Every time I void I take it into my hand and am reminded that I am not normal."

"I don't think that there is a day that goes by that I don't wish that I was able to have an erection. My wife and I don't talk about it and I have never discussed it with my friends, but it is on my mind."[3]

One more final comment: my own. "My penis is just dead. I can't exercise it. It doesn't move. It doesn't respond. It just hangs there. It will take a long time to be able to live with this."

Since I had known nothing about impotence, I did more searching. I learned that it remains one of the last few medical/psychological issues rarely discussed in public. A friend, aware that I was researching the topic, sent me, without comment, a clipping that began, "Probably nothing brings a man's self-concept so abruptly into doubt as the experience of impotence. Perhaps it is for this reason that so many of this country's 10 million or more chronically impotent men remain silent rather than seek help."

I thought skeptically, "If men don't talk about this, how did someone find out an incredible ten million might feel some of the things I have been feeling?"

Later I read in the *New York Times* about Impotents Anonymous (I-Anon), a group formed by Bruce and Eileen MacKenzie after he had become impotent.[4] They had discovered that, "There was literally no one to talk to. It's a very personal thing to talk about . . . . The doctors can do the surgery but they can't tell you what it is like." The article told about Joe, a 58-year-old retired steelworker who had become impotent as a result of his cancerous prostate. "It was rough," he said. "My wife would say sex isn't everything, life is more important. She tried to help, but there's no way."

Just like Maryjane's attitude.

"I was glad he was alive and my kids had a father," his wife said. "But a man looks at it differently."

"Exactly," I said to myself when I read this comforting news. If only I had read this earlier, when I had begun to think that my exaggerated preoccupation with my impotence was morbidly perverse.

I had known of the I-Anon group and had earlier attended several of its meetings. The men at the meetings that I attended were more interested in learning about penile implants than in exploring very deeply what their impotence meant to them. So I had to search deep within myself to understand further its more subtle meanings to my maleness that had not yet been dredged up by my first revelation.

How had I felt about my body and about myself as male? I had always felt good about my body. I am tall, lean, and muscular. My shoulders don't sag; my rear end is not flabby. I have strong facial features and a firm handshake. In two unshaven days, my beard grows heavy and black. I still have predominantly heavy coarse black hairs on my chest. I look male.

I also act male. I walk and talk like a male and am active, assertive, forceful, intrusive. Maryjane says, ambiguously, that even my mind is male. In court, I aggressively probe, though rarely attack, witnesses. I will interrupt, force answers, suddenly shift to seemingly irrelevant questions to get under a witness's skin. But I am not macho. I have never questioned my masculinity, never felt driven to overcompensate for some doubt. I am content not sporting a beard, though I think my moustache does lend a slightly passionate aura.

I don't think of myself as a typical male, whoever he is. I don't drink beer "with the boys" nor do I spend hours watching football on TV or playing poker. I don't have time. If I did, I'd want to be with Maryjane. Though I know that some of my own reactions and peculiarities may not be typical of my sex, I have never doubted my maleness and have never wanted to be female.

Anyway, I felt at home with my male body and kept it in shape but not compulsively. I enjoyed being nude, swimming nude, even looking at myself nude, just as I enjoyed watching my cock's first flight. I enjoyed stretching my entire body into an erect cock! I was proud of what

I was. I guess in a way I loved my body.

Certainly one cause for feeling so good about my body was the healthy size of my penis; I never once felt ashamed of it. In school, I wondered what kind of boy I was to enjoy comparing it to those of others, until I saw other boys, later college students and even elderly men in public urinals, surreptitiously glancing at the penises of other males. Other males also seemed to be fascinated with penises, took pride in them, made all kinds of crude jokes with each other about the length of other men's cocks, and even desired longer ones. Shere Hite reports that, "most men wished over and over that their penis could be just a little larger. . . . Only a few men were not concerned with size or felt they were just right."[5]

Fascination with erections has been so widespread throughout history and among different cultures that I have wondered if there is not some universal biological basis to male pride. Such fascination goes back thousands of years. A drawing on one Egyptian Pharaoh's tomb shows a man with an erection at least a foot and a half long. Then there are those famous Greek vases, Pompeian graffiti, Indian phalli and temple sculptures, photographs collected by the anthropologist Edward Evans-Pritchard of nude Nuer males with extraordinarily long cocks, and on and on. The owner of an Amsterdam porno shop exploited male preoccupation with erections by placing a poster in his window that pictured an African who had a two-foot-long hard penis tapering and circling back to his chest. I was intrigued. How did he urinate without getting wet? How could he have sex? What a price men would pay to have long pricks.

This historical male preoccupation persists today, for I discovered that one of the most frequent questions asked by impotent men who want penile implants was, "How long will my penis become? Can you make it bigger?" I asked these questions too. Disappointingly, the answer is, "No longer than it was before and probably shorter." Even Dr. Paul seemed interested. When I asked what I would do with an implant that gave me a permanent erection, he said, "Well, you could enjoy being more fully packed than other men when wearing your bathing suit." That appealed to my vanity!

I now accept my interest in other penises, particularly erect ones, as I have my interest in my own penis and in womens' breasts (though it offends Maryjane when I glance at others' stellar examples). After 30 years of marriage, Maryjane still undresses with her back to me and when I try to look, she hides herself even more modestly.

My anxiety about how my penis had shrunk persisted for more than a year. It was not my imagination. Maryjane agreed. One week, in my "adolescent" phase, I even kept a tape measure nearby to keep track of any hope. Once when it crept to four inches, I excitedly called her to come and see, not quite a request that appealed to her, I noticed. I began to realize how troubled I was by my loss of an erection about two months after my operation. For months thereafter, I dreamt of having foot-long, even longer, erections. Six months into my recovery I had one dream that illuminated my less conscious self as well as our differing interpretations about my erections:

> I was in a car. I had a long flagpole that I tried to screw onto the outside of the car. I got it upright. It was very tall but I was not able to keep it up. I then noticed that up above were electric wires so that if I moved the car I could get the flagpole in touch with the wires. I was unable to keep the pole upright and eventually had to let it lie flat on the ground.

I thought it told me not only how much I still wanted a long cock but also that not until I could get the "pole" upright would I feel a charge, some sexual desire. The dream told me I failed in my experiment to get it up, perhaps representing a beginning acceptance of my impotence. Was it also telling me that at this time an artificial implant might enhance my desire?

Maryjane's reaction was quite different. She interpreted the electrical wires as a symbol of death; if I had another erection I would get "electrocuted." To her, not having an erection was a sign that the prostate had really been removed and that I no longer had cancer—a possibility I had never thought of, since I didn't feel upset or disturbed by the dream. Up to this point, I had been much more concerned with having lost my cock than with the possibility of dying.

In some deeply irrational way, then, I feel males who have big cocks are more male. And while I am aware of the folklore that big erections can better satisfy women, I must honestly say that that has not been a primary reason for my wish for a large vital cock. My reasons are more self-centered and primitive, I think. My illness showed me, just as those nighttime orgasmic spasms had, how deeply imprinted in my pelvic reflexes is the need to physically thrust, to drive into, to "plough fields," to move almost violently into another. I was shocked to discover a "rapist" in me. I am uncomfortable writing that, but innumerable times while loving Maryjane, I would playfully act like a bull or stag and pretend that I was ferociously loving her. Somewhere deeply buried in my groin is a forceful aggressive power that only emerges when I fully submit to my own biology. Perhaps because I've sensed unconsciously the potential of such power, I've always been very tender and considerate with Maryjane, never rough, demanding, or exploitive.

To me, it is only a large sturdy cock that can plunge deeply. I have always been puzzled about how men with small penises can thrust deep enough to have any feeling of being "inside." Maryjane rebels against such ideas and says that she can't understand them. Exploring my revelations told me that my male way of "knowing" another is quite different from a woman's. I began to appreciate that my cock was programmed to be wildly adventurous, eagerly assertive, forcefully intrusive, sensuously physical in contact with another. Another part of me was built to be tender and caring, so my "pure" maleness has never been fully unleashed. Not having my cock to thrust with for months and the wild flashes of desire that possessed me when I was doing my daily exercise of thrusting through my bedroom door revealed the depth of the hurt to my body's maleness.

Impotence equals a cock humbled

Removing my catheter made me begin to confront my emotions about my cock's apocalypse, a calamity my subconscious and I spent months denying. The first denial occurred 27 days after the operation. I was taking a hot bath treatment, lying back, eyes closed. I could feel my cock rising firmly. Exhilarated, I looked and saw my dead penis. I touched it because I didn't believe what I didn't see. For months, particularly when I was drowsy, I felt my penis to be hard, only to discover I was hallucinating. I know now exactly what a person feels like who has had a leg amputated but who still "feels" that it is present and may even try to walk on it.

The second denial occurred shortly afterward and continued for months. I began to have vivid dreams. There was one in which I had a magnificent hard-on and I felt I was myself again. I told Maryjane the next morning that I had a wonderful dream. She immediately guessed what it was about.

The third denial was more conscious. Despite the fact that a radical prostatectomy and radiation made it almost 100 percent certain that I was permanently impotent, Maryjane maintained her faith that given the passage of time my potency and orgasm would return. I didn't have such faith in "time." Furthermore, I was not going to just lie back and submit to the apocalypse. I decided to experiment to bring back my erection. Reasoning that if the nerves had been cut maybe they would regenerate, I asked Dr. Paul, who had had cases in which erections had returned. He said, "There is just too much we don't know about what causes erections." I found this incredible in this day of so much medical knowledge. Searching the urological literature, I discovered an article by Walsh and Donker in which they claimed to have discovered the pathways of the erectile nerves and so were able to perform prostate operations that left 30 percent of the men under 60 potent.[6] Since the nerves hug the capsule of the prostate, I wondered if that meant the capsule could not be fully cut out. For men like me, whose cancer had penetrated the capsule, preserving one's potency might be at the expense of increasing the possibility of cancer escaping into the body. Research on the physiology of erections had in fact advanced so rapidly since my operation that researchers are now confident that they will soon understand the neurotransmitters of erections.[7]

Still, discovering that potency might return was all the impetus I needed. I naively plunged into a rigorous sustained campaign to regenerate my erectile nerves in the area the researchers had identified. Reasoning that I needed a refurbished blood supply to my pelvic area, I marshaled all kinds of forces to the area to shock my system: I endured countless hot sitz baths, whirlpools, and jacuzzis; I alternated hot and cold treatments of my lower abdomen; I diligently persisted with my pelvic exercises; I even frequently caressed and manipulated my groin. I became so tense and sore that I had to temper my enthusiasm.

How else could I get two cut nerves to rejoin? Knowing nothing about nerve regeneration, I tried my own homegrown remedies. I reasoned that if my penis had responded to my sexy fantasies, then I might be able to tingle the nerve still attached to my mind by all kinds of vivid imagining, both self-induced and externally induced by X-rated movies and pornography. Dr. Paul agreed. He prescribed a graphic evening of sexual stimulation watching X-rated films. For the first time I openly, rather than furtively, marched into adult book stores to scan *Playboy, Hustler,* and anything else available. I actually became quickly bored.

Nothing worked. My penis never rose a millimeter. It became exhausted. So did I. Stimulating myself so intensely with so little effect made me fear that what little erotic desire I had might burn itself out.

But I was beginning to accept at a different level of awareness that my proud but willful cock had finally been subdued, conquered, humbled. One hundred and fifty-four days after I had lost my cock, my inner doctor began suggesting compensatory "benefits" from being impotent: I could no longer father a child. This was some reassurance to Maryjane, who was still potentially fertile. I could now sunbathe or walk around in a shower room nude with perfect assurance and serenity that I would never again be embarrassed. We would never again have to clean up messy semen. I had an unimpeachable reason for why I could not "perform." A meager list of "benefits" indeed.

Still stubbornly denying my cock's apocalypse and refusing to accept my muted orgasm, I searched for other keys I had not yet tried. What were they? Where were they?

8
The Second Revelation: Communion with Males

I was twelve. My "gang," eight boys all about the same age who knew nothing about puberty, had been fascinated for several months by the appearance of our pubic hairs. Quite proudly we would show our first hairs to one another. Poor Johnny came to mind. Long after the rest of us had moved on to explore what our lengthening penises and their erections could do, his pubic area still remained undistinguished. The warm, exciting feelings of those months of common exploration flooded back amid my continued sobs. One boy told us about a condom machine he had found in a local gas station. Someone suggested we all chip in toward the 25 cents to buy one. None of us knew what they were really used for, but we agreed excitedly. Since my penis was biggest when it was hard, someone suggested I put the condom on and show them how it worked. I refused.

Twenty-nine days after I had been shaved I detected my first pubic hair returning. Ten days later I noticed for the first of many times cocky young males walking down the street. I became inordinately envious. Vivid imaginative fragments of how powerfully their hidden cocks could thrust brought back a cascade of confused, excited, nostalgic, depressed feelings. I felt twinges of jealousy and thought, "I wish I were they." I thought of their potency, of all the fun and adventures they had ahead of them discovering their cocks.

Bronzed, half nude, vigorously active young males in sexually suggestive poses in magazine advertisements also sparked envy and wistful regret. My reaction? I averted my eyes because it reminded me too much of what I was not.

In midsummer when haying began, groups of tanned, bearded young men would come to town to shop, dressed only in ragged cut-off jeans, exuding healthy sexual vitality. I thought, "What courage! The slightest sexual arousal would bring their cocks immediately out from under their bare covering." And I became depressed:

> If they had stopped to ask me for advice, at the moment I would have said, "Enjoy your cocks as frequently as you can!" I had never really enjoyed mine when I was their age. My final solution for my own responsiveness had been a scrupulous but fruitless effort to control its need for stimulation and release. When its demands became more insistent, I fled into a suppressive Puritan morality and the ideal of being virginal for my future wife and then monogamously faithful to her—ideals more common in our culture decades ago than now. Impotence is showing me how much more I could have connected to others, for I now have too strong a feeling of not having lived the full potential I had for different relationships.

The fleeting wishes of a rapidly aging impotent male wishing to recover the springtime of his desire? Perhaps, but to me these feelings meant much more about the depth of my loss. In her book, *First, You Cry,* Betty Rollin describes how envious she became after her mastectomy of other women's publicly visible cleavages.[1] I felt quite close to her. More importantly, these wistful moments of erotic envy prefigured my inner doctor's "plan" for my becoming a healthier, more whole person. Thirteen weeks after the operation, these moments of envy were my first glimmer of what he had in mind for me, though I didn't fully understand for months. To be healed I had to turn erotically away from myself to reconnect with others, first with males and then with females.

Why did my inner physician point the way through the second revelation? I had absolutely no desire to be an adolescent again, except for one wish, now no longer realizable: to relive my sexuality differently. Today, if I were a potent adolescent, given the changed cultural values about sex and guilt, I could have explored my sexuality more freely. Two complicated erotic themes interwove themselves through months of exploring the meaning of my erection to my relationships with other men: male intimacy or bonding and competitive dominance-submission.

Erections equal potential for male bonding: "My gang . . . would show . . . (their) first hairs to one another."

Our gang reveled in our mysteriously changing bodies. No one had told us what pubic hair meant, certainly not what we could or should do with our budding erections, or what that gooey wetness was that some of us had begun to feel upon waking up in the night. So we could explore only as our bodies guided us. Since all of us (except poor Johnny) had similar reactions at about the same time, we were bonded together in a fraternity of shared but secret erotic excitement. We didn't know it, but we were growing up in a culture that severely censored anything sexual. Everything we learned was firsthand. Fortunately so, I now think; for we never encountered inhibitions, hangups, and guilt in those critical first erotic years. Only when my older brother, on vacation from college, stumbled onto one of my gang's mutual explorations did I learn that I was expected to feel guilty about my erections. My severe judge was too late. I never felt guilt about something that all of us found so enjoyable.

We played countless hours of erotic games. Strip poker was one of my favorites. When we began to tire of our own nudity, we discussed for countless hours the possibility of inviting three older girls on the block to join us. But no one had the courage to ask them. Another time, one boy stole a lot of paper cups to challenge us to get our "things" hard, which was easy to do in those days, and see how many cups each boy could stack on his prick. Because I won, I was later elected to the condom trial. With no conscious knowledge, our bodies urged us to focus increasingly on our penises. We enjoyed playing with one another's. I remember sitting under a street lamp one dark night with a friend from school, who, we had all agreed from his debut in the school shower, had the largest penis of all. That night he suggested we compare. I knew his would be bigger. It was. But I didn't care. I just felt honored to have been invited to the trial.

So I blissfully and innocently learned about one facet of my sexuality.

Our gang had not yet fractured into more intimate pairs. Nor had we dared to invite the three girls on the block, who condescendingly treated us as "little boys," to play with us, even when we could have used them in our endless baseball and football games, or to go with us on our longer bike rides, or to see how many items we could swipe from the local five and dime store, or to join us every Saturday afternoon at the movies.

Then my family moved to another state. The bonds broke. I could connect with no one, for I was the foreigner to the cliques and gangs of my new eighth grade. My sexuality went underground for years. I became very lonely. I never learned how to connect with males, and never felt part of any other group of males, even a college fraternity. So I lost the opportunity to participate in the prolonged collective male search of testing out what masculine prowess meant to most other males. I do have many male friends but, like the friends of most men I know, none is close or intimate. Maryjane is my best and only close friend.

My second revelation showed me the beginning interpersonal meanings of my erection. A deeply erotic current in my nature that I had trustingly accepted had drawn me into many adventurous playful explorations and experiments and revealed my strong need to be affectionately connected to other males. A natural move toward increasingly close intimate male friendships at an age when they would have had infinitely less complicated consequences had been blocked by my family's move. Ever since, I have felt incomplete, even empty, in my relations with males. A significant portion of my erotic life remained stuck in unfulfilled needs for an adolescent chum or pal. I did not feel emotionally free to move into the typically less intense adult male-male relationships. So I have always wished for and sought to have as open, playful, loving, and intimate a male friendship as I have had with Maryjane.

My impotence confirmed what I had been gradually accepting prior to the decision to allow myself to become impotent. I never again would recover the primitive, emotional, utterly open, even wild, erotic kind of male intimacy I had glimpsed when I was 12 years old. The pain of knowing I could never fulfill a very central need for communion caused me to turn inward to understand the meaning of my male-male relationships.

Perhaps because our gang of eight so shamelessly enjoyed our mutual erotic communion, I have never felt conflicted about my eroticism—only guilty about my early inability to control its principal spokesman. In fact, I have always valued the great treasure left by those early years of puberty. The openness to rely on the erotic as a way of knowing myself and another, possibly a more feminine mode of knowing and relating, complemented my more visible aggressive, intrusive masculine mode. It was a treasure because it gave me access to my inner self and a different, sometimes creative, way of thinking about legal issues. I seemed to be able to take a different stance from the conventional in my field that sometimes opened the way to a compromise or resolution that more competitive, adversarial male lawyers had not considered. And I noticed when working with painfully troubling divorce and child custody cases how naturally I could become open, even submit to my underlying erotic stream and flow with it into the inner lives of my clients. They said that I was intuitive, empathetic, that I understood. I think I can feel the less conscious feelings and fears of the conflicted men and women with whom I work because of my easy access to the traditionally "feminine" aspects of my character.

Because my cock had been so responsive to minute changes in my erotic feelings, I had become very sensitive to slight changes in its size. Not until it died did I realize how much I had relied upon it for clues about how I felt about others. Those whom my cock saluted, I felt attracted to, drawn to, more open to share feelings and insights with. I spent more time with clients who brought my underlying eroticism closer to awareness. I thought of their cases more frequently when driving to and from work. My mind became more alert and clearer; though more excited, it also became more finely tuned. I was a much more competent lawyer with those clients I liked. I put more of myself into their cases. Fortunately, my earlier struggle to command my wayward cock had so strengthened my will that I never violated my professional ethic. I never trespassed on the sexual sensitivities of my clients, as vulnerable and even receptive as some were, including a few males reciprocally tuned into their own eroticism. I kept my cock's message to myself. I did learn, however, early in my work not to accept some clients who actually made my cock shrivel up. My energy and talents would react similarly. I often felt guilty charging them for the services of a limp penis. Perhaps I should have had a special "cock" surcharge for those clients who attracted me most.

When I was younger, my cock provided a template for knowing others. After my operation I finally realized why ancient people used "knowing" to mean "having sex with." I was puzzled about why so many of my male friendships were so thin, so bland, so unexciting, so static:

> My male friendships that have persisted have little or no erotic attraction for me. They are not self-disclosing ones that open us to our inner cores of being. They are more outwardly directed, focused on our work, bridge playing, tennis, politics, children, projects. It is as if for me to go deeply inward and be self-disclosing I have to do it with my whole body. I don't know how to put it. It is my meaning of intimacy, I guess. I have to know someone through my body. I was talking recently with a young friend about how to really get to know another. I said I do not get to know another only through abstract intellectual discussion, but also physical activities in which we had to work with or touch each other, contact sports, wrestling, in which I could feel his receptivity and defensiveness, his dominance and submission. It is how I learn much about the personality of my masseur and how he felt about me. It is how I learned about how Maryjane really felt about sex. Our bodies do not lie, much as I sometimes wished my cock would have been less honest.

Since I became impotent that urge to look for closer male friends seems to have diminished. My penis no longer confirms it when I think I might be attacted to someone. I don't feel as erotically engaged when working with my clients. I am beginning to regretfully regard my views about my erotic incompleteness as romantic adolescent sentimentalism, to be left behind, part of my transcended adolescent history.

For four months I had been struggling to understand my three revelations, particularly why I felt so erotically poignant about my pubertal memories, when Maryjane gave me Thorkil Vanggaard's book, *Phallos: A Symbol and Its History in the Male World,* which she had seen in the fifty-cent section of a local bookstore.[2] I was impressed by his scholarly erudition about historical, psychological, and anthropological findings. He confirmed that the meanings of my erection were not, as I said after reading the book, "so odd or perverse or inverse or diverse or reverse" as my conscience had begun to make me feel. To support his thesis, he had appended to his book erotically vivid photographs of phallic Stone Age and Bronze Age paintings and petroglyphs, huge sixteenth-century erect cod-pieces, and so on.

Drawing on such varied evidence, he claims that there is in heterosexual males a "homosexual radical," most clearly seen in youth, but present beneath "the threshold of consciousness . . . in any man, [which] is handled in different ways, determined by our particular pattern of civilization, unfolding its effects in disguised forms."[3] As civilization has developed, particularly since medieval times, he claims, mens' consciousness has narrowed; now males no longer have easy access to the radical's energy and so have become emotionally impoverished. (Maryjane later told me that Jung's concept of the anima archetype is similar.) Had my own intense erotic responsiveness been resisting such narrowing of my own consciousness, putting me into conflict with a society that channeled eroticism so narrowly?

Vanggaard cited numerous examples of societies that valued male-male erotically bonded friendships without posing a threat to male-female heterosexual values. The Spartans, he notes, had elite platoons of paired lovers who went to war, inspired to fight for and create great deeds for each other, without sacrificing their basically heterosexual identity. For the first time I understood another erotic encounter I had had in my early twenties. I had been invited by a good friend to visit him and attend his older brother's wedding. In those less wealthy days in smaller southwest homes, unmarried males shared the same double bed, which I did with his brother the night before his wedding. In the dark of night, he sleepily turned over on me and with his hard-on started to pump on top of me. Silently, almost stealthily. I awoke startled, not believing what I was feeling. Old Faithful responded, of course. I dared not say anything; his parents were sleeping in the room next to ours. The next day, he awoke and with no acknowledgement of his midnight escapade became, I assume, happily married. I remained pensive, uncomprehending. Maybe he thought I was his girl? How could he? He must have felt Old Faithful. Vanggaard helped me to understand better. Another part of my past completed.

I do not have the expertise to evaluate Vanggaard's thesis. But many of his themes were true for me, including the need for loving communion with a male as fully shared as with Maryjane and a richer variety of ways by which to express my eroticism. Erotically, I really belong back in Spartan days. Certainly, no later than the sixteenth century!

More provocative were his insights about the erotic meaning of dominance and submission for males, another incompleted pattern for me.

Erections equal dominance: "Someone suggested that I put the condom on . . . I refused."

The most emotionally disturbing and provocative unknown in the three revelations was that I had refused to put on the condom. I made little progress for months understanding what that discordant note meant for my healing. Eight months after I became impotent, I arrived at the following view:

> If I had put on the condom, there would have been no complication, no puzzlement, no conflict to try to figure out and turn inward to explore my relationships with other males. My maleness could have been encompassed by its demonstration in the first and third revelations. So what remains unresolved and unaccepted is the second memory, the invitation by other males to assume and assert my maleness and power in relation to our common eroticism. And that is what my history has been about since: I am comfortable with and enjoy myself, my sexuality, and my loving relations with Maryjane, with whom I have felt very erotically responsive, but I am not as fulfilled sexually as I have the capacity to be. The real historical conflict that has so complicated my inner life has been my relations with males. They have been the goad, the pebble in the shoe, the dark mysterious shadow. Other men have driven me, made me aware, and unknowingly influenced and frustrated my erotic and work relations with them. But this conflict has also made a positive contribution: my creativity has emerged from it.

Puzzling about it since I lost my potency made me realize that not putting on the condom was the first sign of what has since been an enduring conflict: my unwillingness to compete for a dominant role of power that could disrupt my erotic communion with other males. Because I never resolved this, I neither sought to fulfill a natural political leadership potential, as I have frequently been urged to do, nor created a sustained intimate male friendship, which I have frequently but vainly sought.

Our pubertal cocks were instruments not just of exciting novel erotic pleasure but also of vigorously competitive aggressive power. This has always intrigued me because of the extraordinarily complicated ways these two different pathways unconsciously shaped how I would later relate to others.

Coincidentally, while struggling to understand my relations with males, my inner physician emotionally prepared me for what turned out to be another miraculous coincidence. I saw a public broadcasting documentary on male baboons that showed me how deeply my own needs and preoccupations were rooted in my animal heritage. After what can be viciously competitive fights for dominance, the strongest, most virile baboon's leadership is acknowledged by the other male baboons' sexual submissiveness. Vanggaard also described how the dominant male baboon will spread his legs to threaten the other males with his erect penis. Given my preoccupation with the size of my penis, I was amused by his comment that, "monkeys on the lower rungs of the ladder [of dominance] have penises of a smaller size and a paler color than those at the top."[4]

The erotic and dominance templates have been fused in other ways throughout human history: the Hellenic Greek model in which students willingly submitted themselves erotically to their teachers; the Persian punishment of men found in a harem by stripping them naked and letting grooms and slaves sodomize them; contemporary reports of sexual rape of younger prisoners by older dominant ones; Russian and American competition in building bigger and more powerfully threatening phallic missiles.

Not putting on the condom meant not consolidating my emerging eroticism in the typically masculine ways our society expects. I did not channel my emerging erotic communion and dominance needs into competitive team body-contact sports, our culture's acceptable way for males to "know" other males while testing their positions, like the baboons, in their peer dominance hierarchy. This is also our culture's only sanctioned way for males to be openly affectionate and emotional with one another. Nowhere other than on the playing field can two American males spontaneously hug each other or cry. Separation from my gang and failure to replace it forced me to turn back to my own, primarily intellectual, resources, which became the way I was to assertively compete, achieve, and eventually very successfully establish my position in the academic grade hierarchy and eventually in my profession and the courtroom.

Too-successful intellectual control and dominance can lead to overbearing assertions of power and arrogance, which are not strangers to my relationships with other males. My erection had become intellectual power.

One night, while trying to figure out this complicated second revelation, my inner physician came to my assistance. He would say a word and I was to say every word that immediately came to mind. I was not to hold any word back. Feeling like he had me on a psychoanalytic couch, I edgily but trustingly replied to his surprising first word, "cock," with "hubris, pride, self-indulgence, narcissism, pleasure, power, challenge to gravity, natural law, God, maleness."

My inner doctor working hard again! What in the world was God doing there with my cock? My inner voice did not reveal the answer to that for another year.

I was perplexed that "hubris" and "pride" jumped out of my subconscious first. What was I being told? I felt myself being dragged by my inner doctor to face the full meaning of the equation, "Erection equals dominance." Dominance had preoccupied my mind. Suddenly I realized that I had completely ignored the opposite of dominance—submission, which proud people know little of. Was my devious inner physician forcing me to confront my feelings about submission and the price that I have paid for willful control? The cost of not being able to submit to or receive love from authority, like the young students of Greek teachers did, is to not learn or grow. Could it be that hiding deep behind the façade of my dominance, my occasionally overbearing will, was a need to submit, to become vulnerable to another, to be erotically humbled, to present to authority? Knights of old did this when they kneeled defenseless before their lord to have him tap their shoulders with his phallic sword.

Shocked by this opening, out tumbled many confused thoughts and resistant feelings. My defiant cock had never bowed to anyone. I was a critic of all authority, even of judges and God. The image of Dr. Paul returned; the authority who had been my savior. I had meekly and uncomfortably dropped my pants and bent over to "present" myself to him before my operation and allow him to probe my rectum. When I was more emotionally vulnerable after my operation, hypersensitive to my underground erotic stream, I had become increasingly ill at ease being forced to lie half nude on his examining table, legs spread, while he and a resident probed inside me with their fingers. Had I been uneasy because some universal radical, as Vanggaard proposed, was emerging which I couldn't accept as part of Rich Handy? Did I subconsciously wish to "present"? The thought still troubles me as I write it, but it is apparently more widely shared among contemporary males than I had known. Hite reports that 53 percent of the heterosexual males who answered her survey had been or said they would like to be anally penetrated.

These distressing fragments of thoughts—I still have not pursued them very far—occurred about the time I was becoming desperate about not having found the keys that would unlock my orgasm. To me, orgasm had always unquestionably been the result of thrusting and ejaculating. I was a "cock man." No longer being able to do this left me terribly frustrated. How else could I test if I could still have an orgasm? Kissing and oral stimulation was only a prelude to the real thing for me. Being in a submissive, passive sexual position never had appealed to me; under Maryjane, I couldn't be very active or thrust fully. I had never enjoyed anal stimulation, and no penis had ever penetrated my anus; nor had I ever had oral sex with a man. I had never understood how a man could have an orgasm from anal sex or from stimulating another man. My ignorance was showing again.

Was my inner doctor telling me, in the roundabout way of my second revelation, that the route to my healing was through reliving my earlier wild, playful, exploratory adolescent years, emotionally submitting to and not trying to dominate my eroticism? For other reasons, the route by way of Maryjane was blocked.

I had become increasingly so discouraged and depressed by this time that Maryjane asked if I was considering suicide. No, I wasn't. But I knew I was becoming very vulnerable. I was deeply preoccupied by the thought that, though I couldn't get an orgasm from my now-limp Old Faithless, perhaps I could get one other ways. But how? How could I so trust another to be willing to submit in the playful abandoned way my second revelation suggested? I saw no path to follow.

The last trial

Orgasms equal submission

With little warning, I got a call to see a client in another country. I wasn't sure why at the time, but my inner doctor suggested I take along some condoms. I needed some escapist reading for a long plane trip and picked up a novel at the local grocery store. Its cover suggested that it was about two men. It sure was—an older heterosexual male in a position of considerable power who became attracted to a younger, wildly playful, erotic, and handsome younger man. Well!

Erotically primed but physically exhausted after the long flight, I couldn't sleep. I needed a massage, my usual solution to such fatigue. I asked a bellhop who spoke some English where I could get one. He grinned and pointed the way. "Very friendly people," I thought. On the way I got lost and asked a young man the same question, who fortunately could speak passable English. Grinning, he offered to be my guide. As we walked toward what I thought was a rather sleazy part of the city, Juan told me that he was beginning college but he didn't have enough money for his tuition. "Here comes the touch," I warily said to myself. But it was not the "touch" I expected. He said he was a masseur and would give me a good massage for the equivalent of $10.00. Skeptical, I said I was looking for a professional masseur. Protesting that he was good, he took me to several stores advertising massages. I entered a half-lit, dingy, run-down room where six or seven scantily clad young women were lounging. Only then did I wake up. Massage meant sex in this country.

After several more dingy and squalid encounters, I began to pay more attention to Juan, who spoke uninhibitedly about his life and feelings. Casually, but surprisingly to me, he said he was gay and had been since he was 13 when he had been swimming in a river and got a hard-on watching other nude boys. He had never had sex with a woman, was very scared of getting VD, and sought only foreigners, most recently a visiting young American priest with whom he had spent four days and with whom he still corresponded. Yes, he really knew how to give massages. He had taught himself by practicing on a number of his gay friends. He lived with his family in a very poor rural area, but came to the city to earn the money to be able to go to a local college.

Somewhat skeptically and hesitantly, I yielded to my now-not-so-suppressed playful, adventurous adolescent self and to the voice of my inner doctor. While not strikingly handsome, Juan was attractive, clean, neatly dressed. And he was firmly masculine, not effeminate. So I invited him to go back to my hotel and give me one of his "good" massages. I was a little apprehensive about what I might say if the guards patrolling the hotel stopped us. But we cleared that hurdle.

I locked my bedroom door, turned on some soft music and began to undress. So did he. Something other than a massage is about to happen, I thought. Our hour-long tour of the brothel section of the city had shown me how comfortable I already felt with Juan. I allowed myself to relax, eventually submit, becoming utterly open and unprotected with him. I felt that same abandoned trust I had felt when I was 12. For an hour he massaged me, more expertly and lovingly than any other masseur I have ever had. After about an hour, he asked me in his very direct, uncomplicated and accepting way, "Why aren't you getting hard? Aren't you enjoying my massage?" I told him my cock had died and why. He became sad. I could feel his mood change. A few tears came. I was moved. No masseur had ever felt for me the way Juan so sensitively did. Then he said, "I am your friend," and without asking, he gently but firmly took my penis into his mouth and while stroking it began to slowly but increasingly more intensely bring me back to life. I felt I was being led into a miracle I had begun to believe would never happen again. I had as abandoned and intense an orgasm as I have ever had, though of course I could not ejaculate. A deep peace moved through me, washing away months of doubt and despair, leaving me feeling cleansed, whole, joyful. My inner doctor had guided me through my revelations to salvation. Juan quietly left, promising to return the next day. Before drifting off to sleep, I wrote, "I have just received one of the most beautiful massages that I have yet had in my life: forceful, thorough, silent, deep, exquisitely male but lovingly tender.

As I told him when he finished, it was almost a religious experience."
It was at this moment, if I can mark one, that I knew I could be
healed, for I now knew I had the potential for wholeness again. The
next morning, I said:

> I do not have any sexual attraction to Juan, but I feel I can be
> affectionate and giving. His penis is small, so anal intercourse would
> not risk deep penetration. My penis did not change its size at all.
> But I found I could submit to my first embracing orgasm since my
> operation. I told myself to relax, submit to my body's guidance, give
> in to him. So what I learned is that in an interpersonal relationship
> of uninhibited trust and submission, with no anxiety, but complete
> openness, and with intense stimulation, I can have an orgasm
> comparable to what I have had with Maryjane and that an erection
> and ejaculation are not critical.

Then followed two days of recovering the shameless, erotically playful
and exploratory times of my early adolescence. I wanted to discover
and test with Juan the limits of my erotic responsiveness. How else could
I have an orgasm? I asked him to screw me. He was hesitant, never
having done that before. My condom fell off his hard-on; he was too
small. I had the passing thought that maybe I had been right to refuse
to put on this sign of adulthood when I was only 12. So the next day,
I went looking for a smaller condom in a country whose language I
did not speak. I found something like a drug store, and to the amusement
of the two young women clerks, one of whom spoke a little English,
demonstrated what I wanted, since neither of us knew our respective
words for "condom." After showing me rubber gloves, then a suppository,
they brought out some condoms. Somehow I managed to make them
understand I wanted one for a smaller penis. They giggled, intently talked
with each other, glanced back at me and looked at me up and down,
tittered some more, and then asked hilariously in broken English, "Is
this son?" Like transcending the anxiety of entering an adult bookstore,
I was now beyond being embarrassed by this public purchase of the
condom I had refused to buy and wear when 12. I had completed another
phase of my youth. However, as soon as Juan put it on, his cock became
limp. Characteristic of him, with no embarrassment or shame or defiant
machismo, he accepted that this was not his way.

My gift to Juan was my own playfully exploratory massage, to which he willingly submitted so trustingly, so innocently, I again felt like I did when I was 12 and no self-conscious barriers of inhibition, guilt or shame got in the way of sharing communion with my gang. When I finished, he said simply, "That was good." I too felt warm, good, excited, and even awed, by the miracle of healing my inner doctor had led me to. Juan taught me the grace that comes from trusting submission.

I gave Juan his college tuition. He wanted to share addresses. But a part of my past had come to a close. I gave him a long, deeply grateful hug, knowing we would never be able to see each other again. With tears in my eyes, I watched him walk out the hotel past the guards. It had to be that way.

I then decided to test my recovered hope with a woman. At a hotel in another part of the country to which my business took me, I learned that the hotel itself provided masseuses.

She arrived on time. Attractive, somewhat plump with large breasts, she was decisive, in-charge, very up-front. Much to my momentary surprise, she immediately told me in excellent English to take all of my clothes off, which I did unselfconsciously. Her Swedish massage was firm, occasionally rough, not too subtle or exploratory; very different from Juan's. I felt no relationship. After about half an hour, she asked if I might want her "special services." I asked what she meant. She would not say. So I lapsed into silence. She asked again, only more insistently, and increasingly more explicitly. Finally, she asked me obliquely if her massage was making me sexy. She had been monitoring my unresponsive penis throughout. Would I like a breast massage? I told her I was impotent, pointing to my 18-wire-staple scar. I was still hoping a miracle would occur. Did she have the magic to make my penis rise? We hassled about her price, which was exorbitant, given Juan's expectations. She persisted until I submitted, curious to see what she might do. She stripped, tried to arouse me by sucking my nipples, dancing her breasts in my face and over my body, but she refused to "play orally," as she called it. My limp penis felt nothing.

I kept my eyes closed, not wanting to look at her. I was not responsive to her various blandishments, remaining very immobile, even passive. This bothered her and she kept asking, "Why don't you look at me?

Why don't you touch me?" I said that I was tired, enjoyed being very quiet, and wanted to remain faithful to my wife whom I loved. She lost interest in her ministry and began to ask all kinds of questions. "Yes, I would tell my wife." "No, I have never been unfaithful to her by having sex with another woman." Long pause. She repeated my answer and then said, "You're the first man I've ever known like that." Then, quite wistfully, as if musing to herself, she said, "I wish I could find a man like you who would be so honest and faithful." I didn't feel quite like that at that moment. The thought of Maryjane had just returned. As my masseuse dressed she said she could send up another woman to give me a "blow job" if that would help me. But I had learned what I wanted to know. The way had become open now to understand my physician's third revelation.

I knew now that my first and second revelations had become part of my past. The gray depressive fog in which I had been living for months began to lift. I called Maryjane the next day to tell her I had a miraculous surprise for her. I returned to her excited, feeling really alive for the first time since the operation.

Several weeks later, I reflected about the meaning of my experience with Juan:

I feel he was the signal event that enabled me to expand the circumference of my space with Maryjane to reinclude the directly sexual. Juan helped me to confirm that I still had the capability for a fuller orgasmic experience than I had been able to have by myself. I seem to have approached a new phase of healing. And I am almost ready to say I have recovered by accepting my impotence. I find I can now live with it, for the more fundamental erotic side of my being, which I had not known would be in jeopardy when we made the decision for surgery, remains intact. An underlying nagging worry those first postoperative months was what had happened to my orgasmic responsiveness. I had to return to my adolescent self to feel free to explore my sexual potential. It is as if I am recapitulating in this healing process my own developmental history—relying on earlier-explored ways of rediscovering or regenerating myself.

It is interesting that I think of myself as recovering sexually, though I remain as stubbornly impotent as I have been for eight months now. I do have recurring feelings that I am having an erection, and still have the sensation of being hard at times. Am I scaling down my hopes and expectations? I have tested the limits of my arousability, removed much of its ambiguity, and am ready to move into a more direct sexual relation with Maryjane, accepting its inevitable frustrations. Although I am not as upset or depressed by my impotence, I still dream of having big, fat, healthy erections and sexual relations. But now the issue is not the uncertainty of what I am capable of. I am like that adolescent who has gone through that experimental testing phase to discover his reactions, what excites him, what his feelings are, what turns him off, how quickly he can become erect, how quickly his erection subsides.

Now the issue is less a self-discovery than a management process: how to find ways to bring some gratification to both of us at the level at which I am now capable. It is clear to me that fulfillment has to be through others, for masturbation is too much work for the small amount of pleasure and relief it brings. Again, just as an adolescent is pulled by the greater excitement, novelty, intensity, and mystery of interpersonal sexuality away from solitary self-induced erotic pleasure, so am I moving also. How can I find practical, mutually fulfilling ways to love Maryjane?

9
The Third Revelation: Love and Commitment

"Never again will I be able to give you the present I gave you on our second Christmas together." On that day long ago I had told her I had a surprise for her, left the room, taken off my clothes, gotten a hard on, and tied a big red bow around it. My erections have always made me playful, and I charged into the room like a snorting bull, saying, "This is my big Christmas present for you—always!" She blushed and hastily draped me with a nearby blanket.

The affirmation of my body's erotic responsiveness renewed my trust in my own orgasmic capability. But as an impotent husband, what gift could I bring home to Maryjane now? How could I love her now?

Cancer and the medical treatments had turned me deeply inward for months. My healing body had absorbed so much of my energy and concern I had no desire left to reach out sexually to Maryjane. I had little enough energy even for affectionately teasing her, let alone assuming any responsibility for helping her to secure sexual release. I'm afraid I was too bound up in my own body and mind to be concerned for her.

My lack of discernible or insistent desire to make love to Maryjane worried me for months. By the first postoperative month, I was hugging and kissing her. When I could begin to walk around, I resumed my playful sexy games of blowing on her neck or pinching her, when she would let me, or caressing her legs while we were watching television. My sexy humor returned, and I began to hold her more frequently in bed.

Apart from my generally low level of available erotic energy during the recovery and subsequent radiation treatments, I stumbled upon some other reasons shortly after my last treatment:

> I notice my sexual arousal is not interpersonally focused. I have no desire to sexually stimulate or be stimulated by Maryjane. It is all focused on my own body. I think it is because I don't trust myself in a sexual relationship with someone else. I am staying away from such a relationship because it could make me feel very irritable. It would be painful. My eroticism is not yet freed from preoccupation with my body to be able to give it to another. The fragility of my affectionate demonstrativeness is part and parcel of my feelings about myself. Impotence has shaken my confidence in who I am sexually and what I can do about it. It has made me uncertain about everything.

It is fortunate that my sexual desire for her did not return earlier than it did. Our thousands of earlier lovings had not prepared us to resume loving with my dead penis. My inner doctor knew I had other work to do first. Before I could proceed to the third revelation I had to emotionally rediscover other meanings of my erections: aliveness, sexual desire, orgasm, control, male pride, male bonding, and dominance. Learning to submit taught me that my impotence need not be a barrier to sexual fulfillment, though impotence remained a formidable barrier to reestablishing a fulfilling sexual communion with Maryjane.

My third revelation evoked three other complicated meanings of my former erection.

Erections equal initiation: "I charged into the room like a snorting bull."

Losing my erection told me how deeply and primitively male I was. As many women say about impotence, "A man looks at it differently." Maryjane has said many times, "My sexual needs and my feelings about them are so different from yours." And after hearing about and accepting with forbearance my tale about Juan and the prostitute, she said, "How different my values are from yours."

We had always had unspoken differences in the way we felt about sex. My impotence forced me to bring these differences into our awareness, and in the process I, more than Maryjane, had to clarify what being male and female meant.

No longer having an erection has taught me not only about male pride and dominance but also about male initiative and the embarrassing trouble it can get me into. After all, a penis does stick out quite prominently and immodestly and for a good reason. It is, I believe, neurologically programmed to thrust, to intrude, to move into spaces assertively, even aggressively, and this may help to explain Hite's finding that 80 percent of males said they usually initiated sexual relations. "Almost every man who answered said he was almost always the one who made the initial advance in heterosexual relations—and almost every man resented or felt uncomfortable about this fact."[1] Thirty-five percent wished that women would initiate sex more often. I have never sensed this initiating urge to be deeply etched in Maryjane. This initiating, intruding male way has unconsciously colored, if not wholly determined, how I relate to others, certainly to Maryjane. Especially sexually.

I became very aware of how my intrusive maleness pervasively and silently initiated action and assumed responsibility on our first "honeymoon" following my impotence. Reflecting upon our only squabble, when she angrily said, "I can make my own decisions," I said:

> I move too quickly into spaces, even vacuums. This intrusive maleness. I became aware of how many moment-to-moment decisions I make in our relationship. One morning I enumerated them, somewhat to Maryjane's discomfiture. She admitted she didn't want to use her energy that way. I did not even list all of the hours I had had to take from my work to make the plane, hotel, and other transportation arrangements to get to our destination. I just reported on our past day's adventure.
>
> I had decided when it was time to leave for breakfast; planned the order of the day; decided when to leave for the station; called the airline to reconfirm our tickets for home; made the seat reservations; assumed responsibility for finding a restaurant and making reservations for dinner the next day; hailed, directed, and paid the cab driver; bought the train tickets and found out where the gate was; chose the seats to sit in; been alert to when our station had arrived; planned how much time we had for the visit by checking when the last train left for the city; planned how much sightseeing time we had before the concert began; kept in mind a "map" of the town we were visiting so as to

know how to get back to the concert on time; and on and on.

I was appalled by how much energy and time I had devoted to these aspects of our relationship, to how unthinkingly I assumed such responsibilities, and how pervasively dependent such assertiveness made her. And then by how resentful I felt when she criticized me for assuming a particular decision that I so naturally fell into making, with no seeming appreciation for the freedom my male initiative created for her.

It is not that she is a weak reed who does not know her own mind on most things. She does have strong, if not occasionally dogmatic, opinions, like about the arrogance of physicians, and is fiercely committed to equal rights and to her independence. But in many unspoken and even unknown ways, we have been molded by our biological maleness and femaleness to act in the ways we do. These silent rules and expectations, while helping to keep our relationship easygoing and unselfconscious, became questioned when the biological core cause or its contribution to my intrusive initiative no longer existed. In some way, I am not sure how, I feel that the ripple effects of my impotence are beginning to show up in other patterns of our relationship. She has not once, thankfully, ridiculed or expressed disappointment about my dead penis; only regret, sadness, tears, and the wish that the cancer had happened to her.

I cannot demonstrate that my erectile potency and thrusting pattern shaped my assertive authority. I doubt that they did, directly. But the fact that I am a male, symbolized by that willful capacity, must provide a societally sanctioned way for reducing the initiating, assertive urges my testosterone produces.

It was my impotence that dramatized my maleness in our sexual relations and how deeply ingrained an initiator my cock had been. We both agree that I am much more sexually focused than she. Not infrequently, she has said that perhaps I should have a mistress. But I know her well enough to know that if I did, she would be devastated.

What were our attitudes and feelings about sex that led my inner physician to call back the memory of our second Christmas?

I had always initiated 95 percent of the jokes, 99 percent of the discussions about and 100 percent of the invitations to sex in our precancerous 26 years of marriage. Around her, and only her, I have always been sensitively tuned to interpret and express sexual innuendos, particularly since my impotence.

As repetitive and corny as most of my humor is, she always has understood and gracefully accepted it. She knows me so well that she is as sensitively tuned in to my eroticism as I am thermostatically calibrated to interpret even the most innocent of her comments sexually. I have the subconscious of a cock when I am around her.

Our discussions about our sexual needs and relations have always left me vaguely restless and dissatisfied. I not only initiate all of our discussions, but I also have to keep the conversation going. We do not have playful sexual dialogues, shared sexual fantasies or dramas or reminiscences. Sex has only become a topic, usually too brief a topic, when there has been a problem between us. Most of the time my discussion is with myself, so regretfully I have long had an inner fantasy life barely shared with her. Not because I am unwilling but because I feel it would bore her. She would listen, if I asked her to. But that is not what I wanted.

Not able to initiate and have sexual relations for months after I became impotent disturbed all of the ways I had shielded myself for years from my erotically primed cock's insistent waywardness. What had sex been to me before and what could it be like after my cock died?

Because the cancer and subsequent impotence forced me to review my sexual past in such detail, I have risked exaggerating and so distorting my view of who I am. Sex has been important but it scarcely has been the governor of most of my day-to-day life. My underground erotic stream usually only welled into my awareness and actions several times a week. Most of the time it bubbled along quietly, though occasionally more furiously, such as when I was on a "honeymoon" with Maryjane.

We have been very sensitive to each other sexually. Maryjane was sensitive when I needed sex and she almost never refused; I was to her periods of fatigue and disinterest. I don't feel I made unreasonable demands on her. She never asked me for sex. She was always accommodating, even to occasionally faking interest or having an orgasm. But she does refuse to rate on my scale of 1 to 100 how intense a climax she has had! Since I distrusted any contraceptive method that could possibly affect her hormonally and we found her other methods not satisfactory, I eventually assumed contraceptive responsibility prior to my impotence. I chaffed at how insensitive condoms made me, but no other alternative appealed to us.

I always enjoyed our sexual relations, but I knew, particularly when my eroticism sprayed more furiously into my awareness, I could be much more fulfilled in our relationship. All my years of accumulated frustration burst upon me one vulnerable summer afternoon when I baldly stated my problem:

> I feel that she has never accepted my cock. She has never reached out to playfully touch it, except fleetingly during our sexual relations. She has never masturbated me. She may feel I would also feel uncomfortable. For me, my cock is meant to be active, to thrust, when I am with a woman. She is deeply emotionally resistant to any oral-genital contact. She seldom has taken the initiative to vary our sexual practices. After my early efforts in our marriage, to which she would accommodate, sex became predictably similar. I never felt she enjoyed my adolescent type of playfulness. She has been passive, accepting, accommodating. All initiative must be mine: to invite, to try anything new, to be playful or adventurous. But what hurts me most is that my cock does not seem to attract her. I don't feel she really is drawn to it the way I am to her breasts and her genitals. And yet that is part of me that wants attention. I want others to want my cock, for that is so much a part of me.
>
> Now, I no longer have a cock, just a limp penis that even I find dull. Since it has been my hard cock that has initiated and maintained our relations, now that I don't have one, how are we to connect with each other sexually? Even if I could have an orgasm, and if she could overcome her emotional resistance, probably repugnance, to take a more active role in stimulating me, I know after years of sex with her how inwardly uncomfortable she would be. And after thousands of relations that have more deeply etched neural patterns of initiating-dominating for me and receiving-submitting for her, how could we each feel comfortable assuming roles that have not come naturally before? I love Maryjane and cannot now expect her to violate her own feelings or desires.

Reading Hite's report showed me how very typically male I was, not just in my needs and desires but my complaints as well. Eighty-five percent of the men said they wanted women to perform fellatio. Men "want women to participate with more enthusiasm in the ritual of what our culture has come to regard as male sexuality.[2] . . . Almost every man . . . said that he had to do all the work in sex, and that he resented this."[3]

I had not confronted my own conflict over submissiveness at the time.

My first and second revelations told me that Maryjane was not to be my route back to my lost orgasm. The path lay elsewhere and the miracle, as I told her, was that Juan appeared to guide me along it. Our problem remained but now it was clearer to me. I summarized it this way:

1. I am an erotically oriented, readily sexually arousable person. Eroticism serves as a continuous, low-level background.

2. My sexual desire has begun to return as feelings of wanting Maryjane sexually, feelings that were dampened for months by my illness and treatment. I remain very sexually sensitive and responsive to her.

3. My erection had many more complicated emotional meanings to me than I had ever been aware of until I lost it. It has been much more central to my core emotional identity as a male and how I connect with others than I'd ever believed it to be.

4. My currently reduced sexual desire and impotence are probably not the result of psychic distress or conflict or guilt. My cock has been a reliable, sturdy comrade; I have no history of using impotence or suppressed sexual desire as a way of dealing with conflict. My limp penis is a physical reality, not some underlying emotional trauma.

5. My commitment to marital fidelity has sensitized me to having more erotic male relationships as a way of fulfilling a sexual part of myself that Maryjane isn't able to fulfill. Only with her have I been able to sustain an enduring affectional-sexual relationship, even though it is not as fulfilling a relationship as I am capable of having.

6. My sexual needs are much more diverse and intense than hers. I wish for a much more playful, exploratory, varied sexual relationship. I need variety to unleash my full erotic responsiveness and feel as alive as I now know I could feel. I need to submit to very intense stimulation at this point to evoke as compelling an orgasm as I used to have with Maryjane.

7. I feel more free now to resume our mutual sexual relationship if we can only find a practical way of doing it without frustrating each other.

8. My long-term sexual uncertainty is over whether a penile implant will resurrect to the same degree my capacity for an orgasm as Juan was able to bring to life.

A month later Maryjane and I went away just to be by ourselves; it was on these "honeymoons" that my underground eroticism used to resurface very insistently. It did this time as well. But she uncomfortably rebuffed me, feeling I would only become more frustrated and irritable. She was right. So my eroticism poured out in all kinds of witty—so I thought—comments and a hypersensitivity to any sign of erect cocks.

"What are you writing about?" she asked.

"About our frustrated sexual efforts."

"How I let you down?"

"No, I couldn't get it up for you to let it down."

When we were in the subway I saw an advertisement about where one could buy artificial limbs, and said, "Maybe I could buy a used erection there. What type would you like?"

We decided to explore some sex shops to look at various penile vibrators, sheaths, and solid cock substitutes. I teased her by saying I really wanted one of the foot-long ones with all of the fancy decorations to stimulate her even more. I even designed one in my dreams—a strong sheath that could vibrate into which I could fit my limp penis. With much joking I inched further out of my despondency and began to accept my impotence more fully as a permanent part of myself.

I still had some way to go, though, for I became just as envious as I had been months earlier of the strutting young males whose crotches bulged with a vibrancy I never again would feel.

The sheer diffuseness of my eroticism, the ease with which I became excited, and most importantly, my strong urges to love Maryjane again, led me to tell her that I expected to still be sexy when 75. To myself, I said, "If I live that long."

As our abortive loving showed, we cannot know each other fully if I am not able to give. The cast of our relationship is set by the irremediable fact that she can have intercourse and I can't. My erection is the *sina qua non* and therefore I am more vulnerable to its disruption. That leaves the ultimate decision and authority in me and in my penis's responsiveness, though she as a woman has a host of subtle ways to control the timing and vigor of its acknowledgment. My biological and learned emotional maleness have set some very painful limits to my will.

Maryjane's sexual needs have always been nebulous to me. She has always been shy about describing how she felt, uncertain about what she needed or wanted sexually, reticent about her own earlier sexual experiences. I have remained unsure to this day just what her needs really are. For years, I felt she was deliberately adjusting herself to my sexual desires. Of course, my sexual needs were transparently visible; my cock saw to that. I could not escape how I was feeling and reacting. But Maryjane gave me few visible clues about her own sexual needs. When I persist, she says she is content with our hugging and kissing and playful caresses and my holding her at night. Unbelievable. I insist she must want something more. No! Incredible. I learned from Ann Landers that Maryjane is very much like other women. To preserve contemporary marriages, we need bumper stickers reading, "Have you hugged your wife ten times today?" Hugs, not cocks, apparently are what some most deeply want.

I finally have accepted that Maryjane really may not know how to answer my insistent questions. My emerging understanding of what an erection has meant to me tells me what *not* having an erection may also mean. My questions were driven by a deep, unconscious, *male* feeling of what sex is. My former cock could capture and draw into itself all of the diffused erotic, sensuous, sexy feelings I could be unknowingly having and then visibly stretch itself to tell me in no uncertain terms what it needed. Maryjane had no visibly compelling or consciously focusing spokeswoman for her own diffused feelings.

To make a decision whether to buy a prosthesis, an artificial erection, I had to have some inner clarity about whether Maryjane really wanted my erection back. I think she did but only because I did; not because she had a compelling need for it for herself.

She wants to stay a mystery to me. I think her inability to talk about her needs is a facet of a more diffused feminine eroticism not as easily discussed as my horniness. I still remain uncertain after all our years together about just how intense her sexual needs are and how important my own maleness is to her and to those needs. I have trouble telling the difference between what has always been her willingness to accommodate, to silently, maybe even semi-consciously, adjust to my more imperiously asserted needs, and what her own personal needs are. Her personal self is at times so much identified with being a wife, or more clearly being a mother to Lucy and Pete, that I find it elusive to know what is of her and only of her. She is firm, though, about some things, unfortunately. She does not want to participate in oral sex, though she asks, "Why do I feel that way?"

Erections equal love: "Just for you—always!"

My cock has been the most important way I express my love for Maryjane, though other ways are more important to her. I had not been aware of how silent I had been in talking of love following my impotence, until I reviewed the course of my recovery. Other meanings of my impotence had taken over.

For me, love is giving. Maryjane gave and gave during those scary early weeks and months. I was not able to give much back for months. Preoccupied by a body I could no longer trust, a hapless leaky penis, neutered sexual desires, and an eroding confidence in the full return of my orgasmic responses left little energy free to be able to give to her. After the first weeks, I began to give in little ways, increasingly in the ways Maryjane felt loved. But I could not give in my special male way until I recovered a much deeper trust in my own orgasmic responsiveness.

Love had many meanings for me other than just offering my cock. For both of us, it did mean a commitment to "always." Maryjane early tested my commitment in our intense courtship by pushing aside every effort to consummate our love before our wedding night. I exhaustedly passed the test. But such a commitment created years of conflict for me. My wanton responsiveness and my earlier playful sexual patterns strained my will to remain faithful to our marriage vows. My will prevailed but not with serenity. I have never allowed myself to be tempted and I have religiously shied from any emotional or physical involvement with another woman. So I was not emotionally inclined to rely on a woman other than Maryjane to open the way back to wholeness.

Cancer and impotence have now made me more aware that I had been evolving a more complicated understanding of my commitment to "always." It provided too confining a channel for the richness and vibrancy of my erotic potential. My rigidly virtuous exclusion of any other sexual expression created too much inner strain that must have crept unnoticed into my relations with women and with other men. My commitment to "always" seemed to presuppose that I would feel complete, whole, fulfilled, in full communion, in our relationship. That turned out not to be the case as our sexual relations evolved. I accepted that for years as one of the trade-offs for our mutual devotion, trust, and care. So it was a real shock, when faced by cancer and impotence, to feel so intensely the uncontrollable flood of despairing regrets that I had not fulfilled my erotic destiny before my cock died. I regretted that the sparkle and excitement of my early adolescent self had been so aborted by my precipitous move at the end of the seventh grade; that the potential erotic playfulness of late adolescence had been held captive by an idealized commitment to virginity as a gift to my future love; that I had never enjoyed knowing the erotic responsiveness of other women.

Since my impotence, my argument against submitting was a dispute between my will and the complicated barriers it had constructed, and a long, deeply buried erotic movement rising to claim its long-suppressed due.

Juan and the prostitute helped to clarify the meaning of my commitment to "always." I felt that neither encounter betrayed that commitment. My sexual communion with Juan was only that. It did not evoke love as I knew it to be with Maryjane. So I could part from Juan with only lingering regret. My passively immobile erotic brush with the prostitute showed me how irrelevant sexuality can be to a commitment of love. These are scarcely novel insights to a more experienced adult, but each opened the way to reaffirming my commitment to Maryjane: the recovery of trust in my body's sexual capacity and awareness of how much more fulfilling sex is when it is an expression of love, not just of a body's need for release.

So what was my gift of love to Maryjane to be in the future?

Erections equal me: "I got a hard-on and tied a big red bow around it."

My third revelation pointed the way, not with a hard cock that could actually be felt and on which a big red bow could be tied, but with what that hard cock now stood for: all the meanings of my erection in all of their nakedness and transparency; complete openness of my maleness and its needs; what wholeness had to be for me as a male.

Several days after my healing experience with Juan, I described the gift I could bring to her this way:

> The third revelation, which I have not dealt much with yet, points to an exhibitionistic mode of sexual connectedness, not of direct sexual intercourse. Why? I wonder if it points beyond just sharing a cock I no longer have to sharing with her all that I am, with no suppressed desires, adolescent longings, or frustrations; to being utterly open with her, even about these sexual adventures with Juan and with the prostitute. I don't know how much my former reluctance to share my frustrations was a reaction to my feeling she again would throw a blanket on them to hide me from her, or how much she might feel my straying thoughts and desires might be a betrayal of her. I have more trust now in our love, probably because I can trust myself more now. I know I love her. I know I don't want to lose her. I know that this cancer threatens to separate us in the future. So I need to be as whole as I can be with her now, for it will be acting out of that wholeness that will be my best defense against future cancer. My gift is to be as whole as I can honestly be.

Just what did it mean to be as whole as I could be nine months along the path to healing? My meditations had taught me how male I was. My first and second revelations were now behind me; revelation three still left me feeling incomplete. Was my inner physician telling me that to become a whole male I needed another cock on which to tie a big red bow? I wasn't yet sure. My sexual urge was becoming stronger. By unspoken agreement we had no sex; Maryjane seemed content, but I certainly was not. I was becoming increasingly restless, impatient and irritable. My daydreams began to roam, but to be fulfilled they needed a cock.

How does one go about getting a new cock? Typically, for months I searched everywhere to educate myself about penile prostheses. I quickly discovered not only more ambiguities but also many unknowns, particularly about immediate and long-term emotional effects of prostheses, which I obviously had become most interested in by this time. Urologists seemed to be more interested in the mechanical properties of their technological marvels rather than in their emotional effects. With only an occasional exception, psychologists seemed to have ignored the effects of artificial erections on the male psyche altogether, even though there are ten million of us who might benefit from them.

Dr. Paul began my formal education. There are two primary types of penile implants: a mechanical inflatable pump, consisting of a reservoir inserted in the groin that leads to two cylinders placed in the copora cavernosa of the penis, the spongy area that absorbs blood to make the penis hard. The fluid is forced from the reservoir to the penis by a pump located in the scrotum. The penis would look and act normal. But it was an expensive and painful operation. The prosthesis was occasionally unreliable, and additional reparative surgery might be necessary to repair leaks and kinks in the tubing.[5] More surgery. I could hear Maryjane's reaction to that.

He recommended the second type, a semi-rigid implant which involved inserting two silicone rods into the corpora cavernosa that could be bent up to give an erection and down to hide it. It was a simpler, less expensive operation and the rods were more reliable.[6]

"What do you do with a semi-hard-on when wearing a bathing suit?"

"Enjoy the envy of other people."

I then searched the university's medical library for all the information I could find, consulted other urologists for their opinions, fruitlessly tried to get some idea of what an erection might cost, and waited for guidance from my inner physician.

I was very attracted to the idea of having a permanent erection. What fun I could have with it. What havoc I could create in my health club's locker room and shower. Who would look? How would they avert their eyes? Would anyone make a comment, like "You have a lot of muscle there"? More likely they would avoid me, thinking I was gay. Then I would have no trouble finding an empty full-sized locker. What about sunbathing on the beach, observing who took a second glance and their reactions? Or waking up in the morning to a healthy sized cock? I read that some men found that their repaired cocks now felt cold to them, since they were no longer warmed by hot blood. But then I thought I would never be impotent again. I would always have my instrument ready. So Old Faithful could really be faithful, defying the ravages of aging. I had other, more morbid thoughts as well, like that when I died, I could defy the conventional world by insisting that I be laid out in my coffin nude with my cock erect for all to see as they came to the viewing. What fun it would be to peek at my mourners' reactions!

My more sober adult self began to utter some cautionary words. How are you going to appear in court if you can't disguise the bulge very well, as apparently some can't? How are you going to feel every time you go for your annual physical? Or when you go to the men's room and the guy next to you thinks you are coming on to him? What will happen to your sexual desire if you have a constant erection of which you are always aware? Is it not the rise and fall of nations that makes history interesting, the advancing and receding tide that fascinates you, the fall that follows summer that excites you, the coming and going of people that you look forward to, the lengthening and shortening of the penis that intrigues you? And how would Maryjane react to always seeing a four-inch prick on you? (A permanent cock would be smaller, sadly!) Might she become so accustomed to it that it could lose the mystery my old cock had held for her? More telling, how are you going to react when you wake up from the operation to discover your erection is now only four inches long rather than the six-plus inches you remember? No used car is as good as a new one!

Then I read that the silicone rods could break in the middle of intercourse. The rods could even rupture the head of the glans and fall out! While that apparently happened very rarely, given my previously perversely unruly cock, I could just see it deliberately embarrassing me, vigorously shaking its head enough to spill my hard-on out onto the locker room floor. I pictured myself down on all fours scrambling after my disappearing erection. Another drawback was that if there were ever the suspicion that I might have cancer of the bladder, they could not stick one of those instruments up my penis to look at it. So I was drawn to the inflatable type. Yes, it was a more complicated operation requiring four to five days of hospitalization. It was more painful. There was more risk of infection. And yes, it more frequently needed repairing, which could mean another hospitalization. It does take dexterity to pump up and release. One man couldn't get his down! What a challenge.

I asked a long list of questions of a urologist experienced at implanting these prostheses. Yes, plan on at least one rehospitalization; it won't last forever, so some day you will have to have it out. No, the pump is not pulled up into the groin when the scrotum shrivels up in the cold. No, it does not alter the orgasm. Yes, you will be aware of it for weeks until you adapt to it. No, your penis will never again get bigger on its own, for to insert the cylinders some of its spongy blood-absorbing material must be scraped out. Yes, you can make your penis elevate to any angle you wish (big plus!). No, it does not alter the sensitivity of the glans. Yes, you can continue to masturbate.

"What does this marvel cost?"

"I don't know. The hospital takes care of all of the costs. I guess about $10,000."

That was an unexpected jolt.

"There must be a warranty for that cost?" I felt I was buying a new car.

"Yes, a five year reducing one."

But, I found out, it doesn't include the labor.

How did I feel? Outraged. Furious. This was robbery—$10,000 just to get my erection back, when two cancer operations plus the radiation that saved my life cost only $18,535 in 1983 dollars. Exploitation of an impotent man's vanity and psychic vulnerability! Just out of spite I wasn't going to allow myself to be gouged like that. The next time I looked in the mirror at what I had left, I continued my search.

I began to shop around, calling various hospitals, even the companies that made the devices. The hospitals' mark-up on the implants varied from 30 percent to 100 percent. The urologists varied only by several hundred dollars in their fees. Collusion. Operating time for the inflatable was less than an hour and a half. Surgeon's fees, incredibly, ranged from $2,100 to $2,500 for 83 minutes. More adrenalin. The hospitals could not tell me their costs, except that they varied several hundred dollars a day per room.

I complained about the costs. The reaction was universal, "You have insurance, don't you?" That made me even more furious. Then I thought of the exorbitant malpractice fees surgeons were forced to pay because of the efforts of some of my legal brethren.

I figured that if I needed to be rehospitalized for one repair job and then eventually had to have it taken out, the total cost could well reach $25,000 to get my erection back. Now I had always felt very attached to my cock, but my practical Puritan conscience quickly did some figuring to see if he was worth such inflated costs. Two orgasms a week for 50 weeks a year, with two weeks vacation off for recuperation, for say 15 years gave me 1,500 orgasms. I figured this was as realistic a projection as that of the government's estimates of its future gross national product. After all, the relative amounts involved were similar. Give or take a few dollars, each orgasm would cost $16.67, not including lost interest charges. Given my frugal character, I relished the challenge of getting my money's worth. Maryjane blanched when I reviewed my financial program! She became even less enthusiastic than before.

The financial costs did not turn out to be the critical issue in my decision. What were my feelings about wholeness now? I summarized them this way:

> The research says an implant reestablishes a man's self-confidence about his maleness. I don't care how others judge me in terms of maleness, so I don't need an erection to reaffirm a societal definition of what I am or should be. A new cock may increase my sexual fulfillment and would certainly enable me to increase Maryjane's. But if we do not increase the frequency of our sexual relations, is it worth the cost to her? Not just the money, but the risk of surgery. She is so busy, fatigued much of the time. We had been having fewer and fewer relations several years before the cancer. Would my refound potency put her under greater strain and possibly create resentment? Would I want an erection even if we had no further sexual relations? Yes, I think so. For I could then still enjoy masturbation, which has been losing its appeal these past months, given the amount of work and minimal enjoyable payoff a limp penis seems to provide.
>
> I feel I am not ready to make the decision. Emotionally, I would like the inflatable implant since I can control it and thereby get all of the advantages of the semi-rigid without its potential embarrassments. It will expand my cock's girth. Rationally, I should opt for the semi-rigid because of its cost and simplicity. But it is the emotional effects I want to feel comfortable with.

Two weeks later I felt ready to decide. My third revelation was now behind me. I decided to get an inflatable implant. I felt good. It was the right decision to make. I was more than my erection, much more. But my erection was me emotionally. I would be almost a whole male again, able to love Maryjane again in my special ways. Several years later I read that in contrast to the semi-rigid implant, more recent inflatable versions had fewer mechanical problems[7] and provided greater sexual satisfaction to women.[8] Men with inflatable prostheses reported more frequent orgasms and more frequent sexual relations—even promiscuous ones—as well as more favorable effects on their marital and sexual relationships, satisfaction with the appearance of their penises, and positive moods since receiving their prostheses.[9] Some fringe benefits of my new technological cock were also important. Never again would I have to worry about my cock's frisky independence, for I would now be in control. I could even let Maryjane know just how sexy I was by adjusting its angle. A refurbished cock would continue to complicate my life in a pleasurable way. It would keep open the possibility of new adventures and dilemmas, thereby enriching and enlivening me and so encouraging me to grow more whole. Hopefully these added benefits would help me to stay healthy long enough to enjoy our three male grandchildren as they struggled with the emergence of their own sexuality.

One year after my cock had died, I told Maryjane that I had found the answer to my question, "How can I love you now?" She impulsively replied, "That is a sexist question. I feel you love me. I am content." Months earlier, when I had begun my search for information about implants, she had urged me to wait a year before getting one. She had been not only fearful of a third major operation on my abdominal-genital region within a year but also hopeful that my erection would return, a hope that I had still been assiduously working to fulfill. Now she again urged me to wait another year. I sensed she had other reasons but they did not become clear until later.

Could I wait another year? Physically, I almost felt like my old self, except that I had little stamina. I was becoming more sexy. I felt that living with impotence for another year could create so much more strain that the surgical risks were outweighed. Another year without sex might well lead to accepting our relationship as it was. My sexual desire might wane, not having any satisfaction. I was a believer in the view that if an organ was not used it would atrophy. The longer we abstained the more difficult it might be to resume our earlier patterns. I was the vulnerable one. Our continued affectionate loving left her content, but not me. I could continue to rely on my own efforts, but that was too solitary and not very satisfactory. I might be tempted to return to seek the kind of sexual communion felt with Juan, only deepening earlier patterns I had begun to move beyond. Anyway, just how many more years did I have left to enjoy and fulfill my still-surging eroticism?

Maryjane persisted in her concern. I became irritated by her hesitancy. I thought my arguments were logical and reasonable. I had accepted and transcended my impotence. No longer preoccupied or depressed about Old Faithful's demise, I could even joke about it with her. I was enjoying exploring the limits of my refound orgasm. And I thought I would be able to accept my new technological cock without making invidious comparisons to Old Faithful's sterling attributes. In fact, it would be even more dependable than he could possibly have been as I became 60, 70, and, hopefully, 85 years old.

At this time of decision, my inner physician intervened, demurring, as was his style, ambiguously. He sided with Maryjane. For reasons not clear to me at the time, he felt that I was not far enough along the path of understanding and accepting the meaning of my cancer to get my resurrected cock back at this time.

I heard Maryjane's unspoken fears and my inner physician's warning. So for two more months my trial continued as I continued working on another concurrent phase of my healing.

Part IV
Meditations on Mysteries

That there was a natural course to the healing process became even a stronger conviction as I neared its end. Learning how to adapt to each new phase, whether recovering physically, mastering my incontinence, or accepting my impotence, seemed to follow a familiar path. Each phase shook me, forced me to turn deeply inward to understand what was happening to me. Eventually, I became less absorbed in myself and turned outward to become involved with others and with my work. Each phase forced me to alter myself: my ways of living, views of myself, my relationships with others. But not until such new ways of adapting to each phase had been tested and tested again did I feel more confident, freed from that phase's claim on my energy and enabled now to complete the healing of other phases.

Not until several years after my healing had been completed did I sense that a similar pattern had occurred in the sequence of phases. Taken as a whole, the phase of recovering from the operations had been a deeply self-centering experience. The phase of understanding my own evolving sexuality led to reestablishing my relationships with others. Nearing the end of that phase freed me to face more directly the central issue of my illness, the threat to my life that cancer had been and might still be. My inner physician led me to reexamine my most cherished values and meanings. Very reluctantly and with great resistance I was forced to answer his question, "Had my cancer been not just an illness of my body but also of my relationships and soul?"

The path of healing, by now very familiar and well-trod, led me to examine three mysteries: dying, transcendence, and resurrection. What I discovered about myself has yet to be tested. Until I am so tested, my answers remain a mystery.

10
Dying: How Do
I Say Goodbye?

In their book, *Never Say Die*, Shapero and Goodman write, "The threat of breast cancer must be realized as a threat to life—not a threat to femininity. We must be honest. And we must reorder priorities."[1]

I have had great difficulty thinking about my death. When I do, my mind wanders away, even flees, avoiding the threat that cancer represents. Why?

One reason is that even now, the thought that I have had and may still have cancer remains unreal. I felt great before two people identified my cancer from some stains on a slide. No lump, no running sore, no bleeding stool, no pain, no gut feeling of the threat. It's just damn hard to summon the energy, the will, to face honestly what hasn't been felt emotionally.

Another reason is that I found it easier, somewhat paradoxically, to explore the meaning of dying than the meaning of my actual death. For months, the real threat to my emotional well-being was not cancer and the increased possibility of a much earlier death, but the alleged cures and their consequences. Incontinence and impotence led to the dying of some core meanings to my life, but I had not consciously felt death's imminent presence. Only some glimpses, some dreams, some shadowy anticipations of darker demons I had kept from awareness for months.

Not surprisingly, dying and death do not appeal to me. It is not just that I deny the finality of death. As I finally decided, after many fruitless months of wandering thoughts about my death, I just did not have the empathic imagination to feel cancer's threat to my life. Or the courage to confront it.

So why did I write this chapter? Despite my denials, I know I have been touched by death's clammy breath. Rationally, I know that the portents of those microscopic stains and of medical experience must be faced. More importantly, I have felt death's cold breath postoperatively in my hidden prolonged depression, my vulnerability to tears I could not release, the silent mourning of my losses, the death of my cock, the last "goodbye" to my children and Maryjane, and in my changing view of death

Depression's hidden undercurrent

"Mr. Handy? Dr. Paul. Your biopsy report came back. Of the three samples I took, the lab reports one has a malignant growth."

"You mean cancer?" I asked incredulously. . . . "What is the treatment for cancer?" I didn't say "cure," not really believing there was a cure. My gut reaction was that cancer meant pain and death.

Death's first chilling touch. Though upset and anxious, my disbelief in the pathologist's report protected me from the immediate catastrophic emotional effects of identifying cancer with imminent death. And when Dr. Paul told us that the cancer had not spread and that I was cured, death as a fear dropped out of my conscious mind. But not out of my unconscious mind! Not until three weeks after my prostatectomy did I have a glimmer that a foreboding dark undercurrent was restlessly moving within. On Easter Sunday I wrote, "I am really quite low. There is no resurrection for me. I feel very pessimistic." Not until three months later, shortly after my radiation treatment, did I finally acknowledge that I was caught in the grips of a depression whose depth Maryjane had sensed for weeks.

Not until six months later, while typing my recorded meditations, did I discover how death's undercurrent had been silently seeping into my daily life those early healing months. I am grateful now that my inner physician mercifully hid its meanings from me until I was more emotionally ready to confront them.

Physically recovering from the trauma that two major operations produced demanded all of the limited energy I had. Those first weeks absorbed my full attention as I sought to cope with my incontinence and physical pain and my impatient urge to get back to my work and clients. To have allowed myself the luxury of being depressed at that time would have hindered my immediate recovery. I just was not strong enough to face death's threat with full awareness.

Although I was an uncomplaining, brave to some but really stoical patient, I had very low, occasionally despairing, days.

Five weeks after my operations, I described my feelings this way:

> The last few days I have been very low, very despondent, partially because I look too far into the future and don't go day-by-day; partially because I am impatient; partially because Dr. Paul said that control of my bladder should have returned by now and it hasn't. I have been thinking more and more of what life will be like if I can't control my urine. I dread the complicatedness.

When I was so despondent, I moodily retreated into my "morbid self," leaving Maryjane alone and frightened. I would irritatedly rebuff her efforts to get me to talk. One day I exasperatedly let slip, "I don't feel like I am living anymore." Her frozen tenseness shocked me into realizing that she heard me say, "I don't feel like living any more." Was I thinking of suicide? No, but I was questioning just what fun there was in living.

I had felt these were quite normal, though delayed, reactions to learning about cancer, having two major operations, enduring the annoying slowness of my recovery from infection and incontinence. But I had not thought of myself as depressed and wouldn't until near the end of my radiation treatment when I could no longer postpone coming to terms with my dead penis.

Maryjane was reacting to the presence of that depressive undercurrent of which I was not fully aware, though I had had hints that something blacker was going on than just the "normal" reactions to the daily ups and downs of healing:

I see my life behind me. I can't throw off of the edges of my consciousness the feeling that my days of living are more numbered than I think. There is something dark looming over the horizon. I don't know what, but in some way or another it is this cancer, maybe it is its sequelae. Every time I see my penis it is a visible reminder that I don't have many more years to live.

Other intimations of something darker within erupted in unexpected ways that puzzled me during those vulnerable first weeks of healing.

I was reacting in uncharacteristically exaggerated ways. Why did pulling out that catheter precipitate convulsive sobs such as I had never experienced before or since? Why could I be so choked by tears when Pete called? Why was I so irritated when visiting friends talked at length about their illnesses and never asked about what I had gone through? I later figured out, with the help of my patient tape recorder, that I needed to mourn also.

As I continued to heal physically and became less emotionally vulnerable, other signs of this black undercurrent uncontrollably seeped into my conversations. There were frequent remarks about not knowing how much time I had left. One revelatory moment came when I was countering the argument of one partner who thought I should not retire from the firm. I impulsively replied, "I feel there is an invisible hand or destiny guiding me to retire now. Who knows how much longer I have to complete other projects?" Maryjane suffered through countless similar comments. "I want to enjoy traveling while I still have time," or "Let's spend the money now while we can enjoy it," or "I don't have much time to complete that project."

In the early stages of healing I was not able to put these bits and pieces of intimations together. But one day the firm's secretary reproved me shortly after her own cancer operation: "Rich, you have to take a positive attitude." I began to realize how pessimistically prone I was to believing that cancer would recur. The apprehension became fixed for months after the hope of complete cure shrank when I learned that some cancer cells had escaped the prostate to migrate to within one millimeter of the surface of its capsule.

The hidden undercurrent was rising very close to the edges of my conscious mind. Dr. Paul's and the consultant's comments that one-half to two-thirds of prostate-cancer patients would be alive five years after their surgery became a conscious emotional reality, but in a perverse way; for no defensible reasons, I felt that I was one of those who had less than five years left. For months I lived as if life was measured in five-year time periods. It drove me to begin to put our financial affairs in order and to set some clear priorities for the next few years. My future seemed gloomy indeed.

Two years later, while on one of my bi-monthly visits to the university's medical library, I stumbled on more hopeful articles about survival rates, a much more complicated topic to study than I had thought. Confusion seems to reign to this day among urologists about such rates. I liked reading that postoperative five-year survival rates varied between 85 and 95 percent,[2] did not differ between men who had had prostatic cancer and those who had had non-cancerous medical conditions or between younger men (like myself!) and older men for the years studied.[3] Such hope was not without tarnish, apparently. For I also recall reading that persons who had recovered from cancer but had subsequently suffered heart attacks had had all of my symptoms: depression, little stamina, and reduced sexual desire. By then I had so transcended my cancer experience that I could pass off such pessimistic findings by telling myself that these were all natural outcomes of being so physically shocked. My forays into the urological and related literature have since told me just how uncertain and unreliable is our knowledge of the outcome of my type of cancer. Whether 50 percent, 67 percent or 85 percent of men with less or more severe cancer survive after five, ten, fifteen years with radiation, surgery, or both, made no difference to me after I had mourned my dying. I had put such uncertainty behind me to concentrate on living as healthily as I could from day to day.

But back to how mourning dying freed me to do that.

Not until I had finished the radiation treatment, reached the healing haven of our summer place, and was about to explore the meaning of my dead penis did my inner physician let me feel the full force of that increasingly insistent undercurrent. I finally acknowledged it:

> I spend too much time just lying in bed. I don't know what is going on. Am I in some post-treatment let-down or just physically exhausted?

I am amazed by feeling so depressed. Inwardly, I need to cry. I feel very vulnerable. I have been curt with Maryjane, distant and aloof. I am withdrawing too much. I don't know why. I had hoped that when I got here everything would be okay. It isn't. I am not reacting as I usually do. I don't feel that same intense, ecstatic feeling I have had every year upon arriving. I slide from one dark mood to another. I have lost my appetite. I have no sexual desire at all. I must be a lot more depressed than I have wanted to believe.

It was the need to cry that I could no longer deny, but could never let myself submit to. As I went deeper and deeper into the death of my penis and then of myself, I would drift off into a nostalgic sadness that not infrequently brought me close to tears. For five months I did a lot of crying inwardly, though not a tear showed. Why? I couldn't understand why I didn't cry, until shortly after Juan healed me of my depression about my impotence:

I wonder why I have not cried since I sobbed that day when I pulled out the catheter. What blocks me? I have felt on the verge of crying a number of times. Tears film my eyes. Am I afraid to give way, to surrender? Have I not mourned fully? The day my parents were killed, I cried without restraint. I have not cried about them since. Am I so built to have a massive emotional purgation with only lingering nostalgic residuals? Did that uncontrollable sobbing drain off some of the intensity of the severe hurt and loss I had experienced, thus freeing me to mourn and allowing the healing process to proceed without too severe disruption of my day-to-day life?

When I returned to work six weeks after radiation, I functioned outwardly as effectively as I had before my operation. I was as fully engaged in my mediating and divorce cases as ever. I could sustain as high a level of energetic concentration during the day as I always had, though I was dead tired each evening for months. Only Maryjane, and occasionally Lucy, knew how depressed I was. But my depression was under secure control by now, partly because I was coming to terms with my actual and anticipated losses and with death itself.

Maryjane has since told me that a study of how patients coped with being unexpectedly disfigured showed that women reacted immediately with emotional turmoil and depression, but men repressed their emotions, gritted their teeth, focused on getting well, and only became upset and depressed much later.[4] Except for the sobbing reaction, that sounded like me. I then remembered how I had consciously pushed aside both the impotence and death issues very early to be able to marshal my energies for healing physically.

A springtime of losses

The second day after I began my talking book I said:

> Didn't Freud once say that a mature, healthy person is able to love and to work? That prescription is too limited. A mature, healthy person not only can love and work but also can separate, surrender, and give things up when it is time to do so. This is the springtime of losses for me. Can I give them up emotionally and feel free to get on with my life?

Some losses I accepted with no regret, some only with much painful work. I accepted some anticipated losses only partially, which is why death has been so hard to accept. Loss and separation provide the opportunity to recapture energy formerly spent on certain interests and loves to develop new interests and loves. Aging and maintaining one's mental health is a continuous process of learning how to separate and lose in ways that further aliveness rather than psychic death.

I was surprised at how easily I acceded to some losses: my firm, for example, which I had begun 20 years earlier. I had never assumed some of the prerogatives a senior partner can assume to avoid pulling his weight, such as selecting only the more interesting cases, or even exercising his power to squelch overt complaining and bickering. Identifying emotional stress as a possible contributor to my cancer helped clarify just how much personal strain my character had unconsciously fomented but also endured in the firm. I also realized that I needed more freedom from the silent criticisms of my partners to practice in the innovative ways I wanted to explore. When I realized it was time to leave, I left a firm that emotionally no longer was my "home" with no twinge of regret.

Sometimes it is harder for a parent to let a child go than it is for a child to let his parents go. Pete had been weaning himself from us for several years by going abroad to Oxford for his education. Although I regretted that I could not attend his graduation in the spring of my recovery, I rejoiced in my freedom from parental responsibility for him. It was time for him to become his own person, and for me to accept his independence of will. I thought I'd let him go, but discovered months later that I hadn't at a deeper, much more emotionally complicated level.

Another loss I never regretted for a moment was my ability to contribute sperm to the continuation of my species. I had never felt that the only, or primary, purpose of sexual relations was to sire children. Even if I had remarried, I would not want to begin a new family. Lucy and Pete had fully satisfied that need.

But having cancer and a prostatectomy led to myriad other losses, many anticipated, that told me for the first time what aging and dying were to be.

My losses were neither unique nor avoidable. It was their suddenness and my lack of emotional preparation for them that exaggerated their pain and dramatized their meanings.

Cancer permanently severed me from the long youthful tie of emotionally believing myself to be immortal—despite all of aging's warnings that I wasn't. I was no longer able to read the fine print of contracts without trifocals, to pick up a concrete block in each hand and carry it to where I was building a summer office for myself, to stay awake to twelve every night keeping up with my law journals. I had still thought of myself as youthful, with unlimited years ahead to complete an ever-expanding number of projects. My cancer changed that. Having had cancer increased the likelihood of having it again. It has precipitously dramatized my mortality and wrenched me out of an increasingly unrealistic view of my body's healthiness and resilience and also of time. I now see how the depth of my pessimism about how few years I had left was itself a measure of how painful this loss of my narcissism had been.

To reduce the likelihood of future cancer, I have had to force myself to reluctantly abandon long-entrenched sensuous delights, like cold glasses of homogenized milk on hot summer days, rich heavy cream on hot oatmeal, and linked sausages swimming in a delicious heavy gravy spread on thick buttermilk pancakes. I was depressed for months when walking up and down the aisles of our grocery store, noting all of the foods that I could no longer eat. I said, "I am dying slowly, giving up one choice after another."

Rationally, I knew how harmful such foods were to my health and how spoiled I was, as a rich American, to even have the opportunity to choose such foods. What folly to spread hamburger grease on white rolls! What self-pity to identify dying with no longer being able to eat steak!

But emotionally, reality was different. And when, as a result of a precancerous skin growth, Tom warned me to not sunbathe, another cherished sensuous delight and anticipated Caribbean vacation to now feel guilty about, I said again:

> I am slowly dying. At what point does living become an obsession devoid of enjoyment? I am dying to my senses: no more sex because I am impotent and can have no orgasm; no more French gourmet dinners because of their rich fat-filled sauces; no more nude sunbathing because of the threat of cancer; no more jogging, which I just learned may increase the possibility of cancer by releasing free radicals; no more saunas and jacuzzis, which draw me like a bee to pollen, because they adversely affect my circulatory system. So nothing seems to be without its tradeoffs! Why live?

For months I aggravated my proneness to become easily depressed, but I have now learned how to tolerate such losses or bypass their negative effects. Now when I walk through a grocery store I don't even see the meat, but notice instead the fish counter. Now I shudder just thinking about eating a hamburger swilled in its own grease. I have become an expert on suntan lotions that screen out the harmful ultra-violet rays. Now I swim several times a week instead of religiously jogging every day.

But the *unexpected* losses caused by my prostatectomy were more painful because they threatened my core values and views of who I was. Believing at the time that they might be permanent losses made me increasingly vulnerable to that threatening black undercurrent.

For more than a year my lack of control of my own body meant far more to me than just that; it threatened my great achievement of control and of seemingly being in charge and master of myself and my bodily and emotional reactions. As I have said, my long battle with my wayward responsive cock had given me a strong will, so to sit in a chair and watch urine drip out of my penis was shattering; to drive 15 miles and have to stop twice to urinate was annoying; to forget to shake my penis forcefully enough after urinating and then feel a spreading wet spot on my trouser leg a few moments later was depressing; to have to rush to the bathroom and not make it made me fearful about being too far away from a john. Damn!

Though my inner physician showed me that I could find ways to forestall such accidents, for months I distrusted my body and my ability to manage it. And I despaired when the months dragged on and I foresaw years of hovering close to johns and carrying a bottle with me whenever I drove, as I still do, just in case I got stuck in a traffic jam. Maybe I am overreacting, but self-control was too close to the core of who I was to not become more and more depressed at its unreliability. Although I eventually regained control of my bladder and rectal muscles and these temporary losses became only bad memories, I now know what aging and dying may be like: the gradual erosion of control of my body and the progressive humbling of a proud image of myself as master of my own fate.

The real battle I fought with my depression was over my dead penis. Actually it had been slowly dying for years, becoming more wrinkled, darker in color, less indiscriminately responsive, less erect. Maryjane and I had been using it less frequently, though I tried to keep its usefulness up to par by masturbation. It required more intense stimulation for longer periods to show its full size and then to arrive. Its sudden death caused the mourning that became the salient focus of my healing. Only later did I understand that mourning my dead penis was my inner physician's gateway to mourning and accepting death. My cock had historically had complicated and rich meanings, so that its death threatened a large chunk, perhaps even the core, of who I was. Ultimately, though, my inner physician showed me that the loss of that part of me was not as central, and so as destructive, to who I was as my earlier sobbing and three revelations had dramatically portended.

What really died when my cock died? What had I believed died that really had not?

I never again would see or touch or be able to use Old Faithful in his familiar, naturally engorged, 6½ inch, leftward leaning, arched state. Nor would I ever again feel semen rushing through me, see it spray, or give it to another. I would never be able to contribute my sperm to some childless couple or to some "spermatorium" that preserves the genetic history of authors who write about impotence. Not such a great loss!

I had also lost my cock's erotic responsiveness, which was always a dependable clue about feelings that I might not have been consciously aware of. I can more easily deceive myself now about how I feel, since I no longer have my erection to reveal the erotic truth. Nor can others now get as reliable a cue from my body about how I am feeling about them. Unless I become more alert to my body's underground erotic stream, I risk an emotional thinning of my relationships and even, as I have begun already to feel, a reduced need for erotic intimacy. Given that I feel most whole, alive, and creative when I am in touch with my eroticism, the death of its most sensitive medium could conceivably reduce my access to its energy.

By having permanently lost an unpredictably spontaneous part of my erotic self, I no longer had to be wary about how my penis might betray and clamorously complicate my life. My former cock could no longer threaten my will. But what a Pyrrhic victory! I am now fully in control of my penis, but am bereft of its former challenge to learn new ways to cope with its straying. So my emotional life could become more constant, predictable, possibly more serene, but less a prod to continued growth and to the exercise of will. Do I really want to be so inwardly serene? Not yet.

It was my *imagined* losses, however, that precipitated months of confused worry and despair. The death of my cock so plunged me into an inner maelstrom of irrational confusion that it took months to sort out my emotions. Despite knowing differently in my more rational mind, I emotionally equated impotence with diminished sexual desire and orgasmic responsiveness. This false equation was only confirmed by ignorance of my own sexual physiology, Dr. Paul's failure to inform me more thoroughly about the sexual effects of the operations, and the postoperative complications that postponed my body's healing and so muted my sexual desire for Maryjane and my orgasmic capability for months.

I became even more depressed when I imagined that as a consequence of not regaining my desire and orgasm I might never again be able to fall romantically in love and have as erotically intimate a relationship with another as I have had with Maryjane. What if she died? Would I never be able to fall in love again? Would I die having sexually known only Maryjane? Sadness overwhelmed me when I thought I never again would be able to spontaneously get as hard an aching cock as I had had for weeks while courting her or when I thought I might never again feel so erotically alive and sexually fulfilled with another. Because it was too threatening to think of losing Maryjane, I mourned this imagined loss by way of my adolescent revelation:

> I never again can have that love-erotic-intimacy relationship with another. The reality is that I have never fully worked through my un-fulfilled adolescent need for an intimate male friend. I have always wished, even hungered, to relive those moments of erotically submitting and surrendering my wary, defensive self to be fully open, not just in words but in actions as well, to another male. I want to be able to love, to be as defenselessly present as I am with Maryjane, to fulfill that incompleted male communion, to share the experiences of my maleness, that had just been emerging with my gang before I moved away.

Thirty-three days before I met Juan, I said,

> I can't seem to put my adolescence behind me. I don't know whether this means that I cannot fully welcome death because I have not fully lived out the inner male communion radical of which Vanggaard wrote.

And four days before,

> I'm having an awful lot of trouble putting my youth behind me and letting go the unfulfilled part of my past. One day I think I have left it and the next day I know I haven't. I feel that empty space now. I have a lot more interior work to do when these nostalgic moods sweep over me. There are more meanings to wrestle with.

And six days later,

To reclaim and then free myself of the hold of past fantasies has been one of the most troubling tasks of my healing. I would not regret death if I had been fulfilled in all of my relationships, including one with a male, as I have been with Maryjane. So apart from struggling with what impotence now means to me, I have been troubled most sharply by how to free myself from the hold unfulfilled adolescent needs have had on my erotic life. Reliving an adolescent desire 40 years later when the body is less responsive and resilient and my experience is so much more complicated and varied is diminishing that fantasy's intensity and may even be allowing me now to give myself more fully to Maryjane.

The encounter with Juan had numerous healing effects: I learned that as an impotent male I could still have as intense an orgasm as previously and so I felt released from depressive worries about having lost that capacity; my desire to love Maryjane sexually reemerged; I experienced immediately after getting my old orgasm back the first creative outpouring of ideas since my illness, which resulted in the genesis and organization of this book and a major reordering of my priorities about using time in the future; and, probably most crucially, I began to reevalute the centrality of my erection to my maleness and my identity.

I wrote after we parted, "I feel I have reached a different stage of self-acceptance. I feel I no longer need grieve for my lost erection." I began to dethrone my old proud cock that same evening:

I have been thinking of my life's balance sheet. What parts of me would I have given up before giving up my alive cock? I certainly would have first given up my left and right small toes, my gall bladder, my appendix, my left little finger, maybe six feet of my small intestine, my hair, my wrinkles and that beginning dark splotch on my hand, my moustache, even one or two ribs, maybe more.

I would not have given up my eyes, ears, any part of my brain, hands, arms, legs, feet, my erratic unstable autonomic nervous system I've devoted too many years to taming, my nose, or my non-cocky penis.

The healing reintegration of myself had begun. I had much to be thankful for. It was only my erection I had lost! What had I been so depressed about?

Had I needlessly been plummeted into my prolonged depression and provoked into urgent, even compulsive, and exaggerated, even desperate, efforts to recover my sexual desire and orgasm? No, not needlessly. My cock had had too many rich historical emotional meanings of which I had not been aware, so it had become irrationally overvalued, as my obsession and despair about its loss told me. Mourning my cock's death by reliving its earlier meanings freed me from its long emotional hold on my view of who Rich Handy was. Given Old Faithful's inescapable death, I had to mourn in the ways I did if I were ever to accept my impotence and get on with my life in an emotionally healthy way. Only then could I become free to accept, love, and be proud of any substitute for Old Faithful that I might get.

I now think that for many men, our cocks are the ultimate hiding place of youthful narcissism. For men like me, the core meaning of impotence, as emotionally irrational as it is, was its threat to life itself. Mourning my cock's death initially substituted for mourning my own death. Could this be why impotence still remains culturally closeted? Is it too close to the meaning not just of our maleness but of our mortality?

Maryjane thinks that for women, losing a breast to cancer may not have as complicated meanings as losing an erection can have for men, since such women can still have intercourse, experience the erotic mutuality of giving and receiving genitally, and create children. An impotent man, however, can't—at least not as naturally or easily. And the emotional consequences and meanings of these differences may be much more central to a man's identity as a male than to a woman's as a female. That may be a male viewpoint.

Mourning my death

Emotionally accepting that I had not died when my cock died paradoxically freed me to begin to mourn my own death honestly. I no longer disguised cancer's threat to my life by focusing so exclusively on my cock's death. However, I could not really feel my own nonexistence. I lacked the imagination to make it a real fact. So my inner physician led me to more tangible questions, like, "When might I be content to die?" "Why did I get so upset when Pete called?" "How can I say goodbye to Maryjane?"

When would I feel my life had been completed, the circle closed? When I no longer desired to see the circus or take Maryjane dancing or see Disneyworld or seek the Caribbean sun in January or go canoeing on the Concord river? When I no longer felt strong urges or needs and found I had nothing to look forward to? When I had purged myself of what wisdom I could winnow from much rich but as yet undigested experience? When I no longer had anything to say or give to others? When I would say, as Churchill reportedly said near the end of his life, "Life has become so boring"? When I no longer had loved ones to mourn?

Mourning was my route to complete what my impotence barred me from ever fulfilling. I had to let go, surrender still-live desires, urges and gnawing empty inner spaces, anticipated hopes and loves I could no longer fulfill:

> There are numerous little bits and pieces of habits and feelings I have to begin to give up, like feeling my cock get hard as I go to sleep; like walking to the john and feeling good about seeing how alive it is; like loving Maryjane on Sunday mornings; like being erotically pulled by my cock to an attractive person; like having another intimate friend.

My inner physician did not let mourning stop, however, after Juan helped me complete impotence's circle. He insisted that I now mourn my own death, my emotional meaning of cancer.

So I turned to ask, "If my final accounting were now, what would I be most remorseful about giving up?" Not my clients, my friends, unfinished projects, or summer sunrises over the ocean. I never mourned these possible losses. But very clearly, it was separating from the children and Maryjane that remained unfinished. From Pete more than Lucy. She had found her way and was developing a strong sense of self as a wife and mother of three boys and as a person in her own right with her own hobbies and career. She no longer needed me to accompany her. Besides, she had a supportive husband to go with her.

Mourning Pete's loss was more emotionally complicated to complete.

Mourning Maryjane's was too painful to complete. I intuitively knew that the route to letting Pete go was in understanding my tearful reaction to his calls. I had no insight for 13 puzzling months. Then my inner physician worked another one of his miraculous coincidences. One week prior to my implant operation, I flew to England to see Pete. The in-flight movie was *The Starman,* in which a planetary visitor, preparing to return to outer space, asks an earthling woman with whom he had gone to bed, "How do you say goodbye?" Just the issue with which I had been struggling when thinking of leaving Maryjane! That I was so moved by her answer and their separation told me that my inner physician was speaking again. I instantly knew he was providing an opening to complete my separation from Pete, and that I had to ask him for his help to free me from him.

A few words about Pete. More gifted and talented than I, he is a resourcefully self-taught person who since he was three has had the urge to rocket among the stars, alone if need be. When we last went mountain climbing together and came to a sheer cliff, hundreds of feet above a small valley below, I had remained a safe distance from the edge. He unhesitatingly, almost brazenly, walked right to the edge and climbed out on a dangling tree branch to get a better look straight down. Looking around he noticed my blanched, tense face. He chided me, saying, "What are you so scared about, Dad?" A question asked by someone who had never been a father who had a son to lose to a cracked branch. He had nothing to lose, being immortal still! Since he was nine, when he secretly built a raft which he poled by himself down a nearby river, he has tested himself against nature's limits. Any unknown frontier or adventure is there to master. As he has gotten older, his adventures have become riskier—to me, but of course, not to him. For he has won each test. So far!

Bored with his college, tired of what he thought was England's insipidly soggy weather, attracted by any place he hadn't been, he had decided to fulfill an early adolescent wish: have a James Bond adventure. He had always wanted to ski the Schilthorn, the mountain that Bond had skied when fleeing his enemies and a terrifying avalanche. When I arrived at his flat, he proudly showed me his new ski gear.

"But you don't know how to ski."

"I'm teaching myself from this book. If you can practice golf with those fake balls in your garage (which I had done one year), then I can practice skiing in my room until I find a hill somewhere." Which is what he did.

For months I had been preoccupied, anticipating Pete's death. But I couldn't mourn it fully, for I could not let him go. I shared with him my fear that he had a suicidal fascination to test the limits of his competence to survive. He felt so differently that I got a glimmer of a powerful life-force—rather than death-force—impelling him. I began to feel greater peace about him. The thought of his death no longer preoccupied me in the way it had before.

Mourning my cock's death and the possibility of Pete's was my inner physician's way of gently preparing me to face my own death and my separation from Maryjane. On the flight home, now able to let a few tears emerge unashamedly but to the increased discomfort of the man next to to me. I wrote:

I feel so much closer to Pete now, not only as a father. If I were 22 again, he would be the close friend I never had. Behind the visible differences in interests and ways of life that have so exercised me these past years, I have discovered how remarkably similar we really are in the ways we think, in the ways we have explored our interior selves, in our perceptions about others, in our unspoken meanings of maleness.

For me, as impotence has shown, maleness centered on my adventurous erotic cock; for him, on his risky, macho adventures with nature. To assert his own independent identity, he had opted for a visible way of life in direct contrast to mine, deliberately shunned my more cautious footsteps, rejected my more conventional concerns about vocation and marriage, and avoided any relationship in which he might accede to his suppressed very affectionate nature, which I knew was still alive when it snuck out temporarily in his caring transatlantic telephone calls and in his few letters signed "Love."

Tales of father-son strains and ambivalences throughout history and in literature are legion. Exploring the many complicated meanings of my feelings about my son have shown me why. Pete was an unescapable symbol of a youthful past that I had not yet fully relinquished. He was a reminder of the boy I had once been. But he was also a symbol of unfulfilled, uncompleted potentials of a youthful maleness that I had earlier rejected or never fully explored, a reminder of the young man I could have been. He had become the hidden repository of unfulfilled talents, suppressed desires and dreams that I no longer could relive myself. I wondered if he was living out some hidden unfulfilled side of my maleness, just as I might be living out an unknown side of his.

So why did I react so strongly to his caring calls? I sensed that despite his visible self-sufficiency, he still needed me. He had not yet found his way. Deep down, he still needed me to go with him. But there was a more hidden, self-centered reason for my tears. In anticipating his death on his skiing trip, I was mourning my own coming trip. His death would be the death of all of those unfulfilled potentialities of mine that he represented. My circle would remain incomplete and I would remain unable to accept and transcend cancer's threat to my own life. That is why I was unable to let Pete go and why I remained preoccupied about but unable to successfully mourn his death.

What could I do to free him of his need for me and mine for him? For surely each of us needed to become free of the other; he to grow more whole, I to accept death with more serenity. Again, my inner physician showed me the way:

> I can see now what I have to give: to be the father to my son that my father had never been to me. To accompany him a little while longer. To be present within his space and not pull him into mine. Perhaps to ski with him on his practice trials. I am no James Bond! To share my own life, the meanings of maleness I have been feeling, to help him understand me, so he has the opportunity to get a perspective about himself. If I am right, we are each living out the other's unfulfilled potential. So, regardless of what his way is to be, hopefully it will be one that will accept his more erotic, giving, life-enhancing side as part of his maleness. And I need to rejoice that I have time left to fulfill what I have not fulfilled in my own past by identifying with his adventurous spirit.

Though I am a mediocre skier, I joined him the following Christmas. I suffered only a mild sprain and shared my three revelations—to his accepting silence.

From the moment I told Maryjane I had cancer, we have both lived under the dark shadow of our mortality. Five years later, we still are on edge after each quarterly check-up for signs of cancer's recurrence. Her fear of my death still lingers in many hidden ways. One evening, months after my operation, I had left the evening dishes unwashed to go to bed early. Apprehensively, she peeked in to ask if I was all right. I once called her to say goodbye before I left for the airport, and she called back a few minutes later to say she hadn't liked the way she had said goodbye. I knew, though—she had had a premonition I might not return and wanted another "goodbye."

Much as I knew I had to try, I couldn't face our separation. I could not keep her in mind. She would fade away only to return briefly in another memory—of when we first met, or when we hiked along the shore, two months after that meeting, planning the names of our first boy and girl, or when I held her in my arms when we heard the news of her father's death.

The closest I came to really feeling our separation was on a transcontinental flight a year after first learning of my cancer. As I watched a movie about a man dying of a fatal illness, tears again came to my eyes. Again my inner physician was preparing me:

> I cannot think of parting from Maryjane without my eyes clouding. I feel like I am in the sauna when my entire body weeps as the drops of sweat—my body's tears—slide down, drenching me. I have the foreboding that I may never see her again. That day of saying goodbye may be sooner than we both know. Each goodbye may be our last. That I can't face. My eyes are so filled with tears now I can scarcely see these words. That is the pain, the hurt that the cancer forces me to feel. I don't want to see it. I force my mind to other memories but I know that last goodbye is but a few hidden memories away. I can't face that last goodbye. I feel empty, dead. There is a heavy, dark apprehension in my chest. I move between thoughts of Maryjane leaving me and me leaving her, but surely that separration is approaching.
>
> I feel myself withdrawing again from meeting Death. I can't imagine

its reality. It is like a damp fog that drifts into my inner mind and then recedes. It brings tears that I try to swallow. I feel fleetingly cold and numb, drawn far inward. My mind is here but only alive to a few inches around me, like to the hand of the man next to me. For the past 30 minutes I have let myself get closer to the meaning of my cancer than I have allowed myself to get before. It is like tentatively reaching a finger or toe out to some new dark space, hastily withdrawing it, and hesitantly reaching out again, only to retreat again, pulled back each time by the black mystery's fascination further and further into the darkness, only to retreat, frightened, again and again until that dark space becomes more familiar, less scary. But I am not yet ready to stay long in that darkness. It so frightens and saddens me. It contains the future I am not ready for, the foreboding fear I have not yet transcended.

How am I to say goodbye to Maryjane? *The Starman* had shown me how—as I said goodbye to Pete. I will hold her in my arms and tell her, "I love you. I always have. I always will."

Transcending death

As was so typical of the course of my healing, while I was preoccupied with one theme or relationship, my inner physician was preparing me at less conscious levels for other themes I still was not emotionally ready to face. Only while rereading the transcript of my taped meditations did I see how frequently he had signaled in shadowy but increasingly clearer hints of what I was to face head-on months later.

Two months before I finished mourning my lost cock, I dreamed of driving on a road that had no end, an endless trip that could only mean death. I next dreamed of being kidnapped by terrorists, escaping from their car, unable to find help because I could not speak their language, and suddenly seeing them turn the car around and come racing back to run me down.

One month later, Death itself appeared more openly in my dreams:

A very stocky but disfigured old man came up from underneath the street. I don't know how he got there but he came up from down below. He was asking for me. I was at my grandparents' golden wedding anniversary. He said he had known them very well. I invited him into the house. He was very observant and noticed some mannerisms of mine, which made me aware of how sharply he was watching me. Was he a psychiatrist? Suddenly Lucy appeared. She was a young girl. She angrily said something to him that I don't recall and then ran out of the room crying. I left to comfort her and to explain that he knew her dead great-grandparents. She returned to apologize to him, though petulantly. I talked to him and then woke up, feeling very good, but wishing our talk had continued. Was Death coming from the netherworld, the world of my ancestors, on a festive day representing the close of a happily married life? I was not defensive or upset. But I feel the dream is a warning that I don't have unlimited time and that I must begin what is yet unfinished.

Thirty days after Juan and I parted and I had completed mourning my dead penis, my inner physician created another small miraculous coincidence that alerted me to the path to take next. I had been typing my tape-recorded meditations for several days. To prepare myself to endure emotionally what I had gone through the previous 11 months, I listened to music, settled myself quietly, and meditated for half an hour or so. This morning I unthinkingly had selected Franck's *Symphony in D Minor*, which I hadn't listened to for years. I wrote afterward:

I seem to have approached a new stage of recovery, for by accepting my impotence, I find I can now live with it. I am now planning how to resurrect my dead penis by getting an implant.

In my meditation today, Franck's second movement pulsated, became rapid, almost rushing, breathless. My heart began to beat faster; my breathing became more rapid. I was empathizing with the music, living its beat and rhythm. I thought of how quick the pace of life is, rushing me faster and faster to death. I felt an urgent beat to living, hastening me onward to what end I know not. But I feel confident that I can meet whatever may come. How I have reacted to the uncertainties of cancer has told me that I have prepared myself for the possibility of and hope for emotional resurrection. This dramatic word captures my greater confidence in my resilience to cope with more immediate "deaths" in the future, like decreasing sight, hearing, or, God forbid, declining mental acuity and imagination. Beethoven was deaf when he created his greatest works. Impotence is a symbol of dying, for it has cut off some modes of connecting with others, but I have a rich variety of ways left by which to connect, not the least of which are my inwardness and imagination, which enable me to populate my life with an infinity of possible inner connections.

And at this moment, I unexpectedly experienced dying. The third movement was coming to a close. I gradually relaxed. My head fell over on my shoulder. I plunged deeper and deeper inward, absorbed in the finale. Everything else was quiet. Even my mind. I felt so peaceful that I felt I was dying. The music stopped. I had no will to summon myself back, though I knew I could. I just leaned back on my rocking chair, breathing very slowly, very deeply—as if, I see in retrospect, I had had some kind of profound "life orgasm."

I had never before read the commentary on the symphony's jacket. It ended with a comment by Gounod, the composer of *Faust*, one of my favorite operas. The symphony, he had sarcastically written, was "an affirmation of impotence carried to a dogma."

Was my inner physician confirming what I had begun to sense, that I too had so exaggeratedly affirmed the importance of my cock that my preoccupation with its death had been carried to an extreme? It was time, I interpreted him as saying, to transcend the death of my cock and begin to put my life into a wider perspective. But what could I then affirm that was not a dogma?

Six months later, only after I had begun to let Pete go and discovered how to say goodbye to Maryjane, I was able to understand the meaning of my cancer experience and so affirmatively transcend its threat to my life.

11
Transcendence

Cock: Hubris, pride, self-indulgence, narcissism, pleasure, power, challenge to gravity, natural law, God, maleness.

Cancer: Death, nuclear destruction, humility, fall, fall of man, "punishment," day of judgment.

These were my immediate and unguarded responses to the words my inner doctor said to me during the brief moment of Juan's ministry when I finally began to accept the death of Old Faithful and the foggy depression that had been obscuring that part of the path toward wholeness miraculously lifted.

I was not surprised that my cock meant "pride," "narcissism," "pleasure," even "challenge to gravity." After all, I had been consciously struggling with these meanings of my maleness for five months. Shaken, however, by my other responses, I refused at the time to explore what "natural law" and "God" had to do with my cock. So preoccupied with mourning its death, I scarcely noticed the next path that my inner doctor had told me to take—to understand my cancer more deeply. A path that led to "humility," "fall of man," and "day of judgment" made no sense to me at the time. Had my striving for wholeness been fruitless? Was I now to be punished for my cock's hubris? Was my inner physician forsaking me now, just as I was nearing the end of this journey? Impossible. He had been my angel of healing and wholeness, not of dying and nothingness. Surely, he had a deeper meaning for me about the mystery of my cock and of cancer.

Meditations about wholeness

What has the death of my cock taught me to affirm? There is a natural law to human growing and healing and God is the principle of wholeness, the goal of all growth and healing. Writing this makes me feel uncomfortable. Too abstract. Too pretentious. I am no philosopher or theoretical physicist, let alone a theologian, comfortable with invisible abstractions. I am only a lawyer, most at home with immediate, resolvable human concerns that I can feel and experience myself. So I turn back to what I have experienced and learned these past four years about God's natural law for humans. Since I deal with law, I'll rely on my professional skill of dogmatically abstracting the "argument" or law, and then document the legal argument from my personal healing.

The argument begins with the assumption that a healthy living system has the resilience to maintain a bio-emotional equilibrium that ensures its viability. Any system is composed of numerous interacting sub-systems, each in turn composed of its own functional integrated systemic units. A cancerous system does not have the resilience to recover its equilibrium, so it acts in ways that disrupt its relations with other sub-systems and eventually destroys itself and other connecting systems.

Emotional healing, growing into wholeness, means integrating and stabilizing or restabilizing a system's or sub-system's functional relations with other systems in healthy ways that enhance the larger system's resilience for acting adaptively again. Physically, healing has its own natural sequential patterns or laws. It is initiated by a hurt, insult, feeling of incompleteness, some disequilibrium. The result of healing is transcendence, a felt sense of completion, of being grounded, stable, whole. Energy becomes freed for new growth; perspective is gained; living feels good, even joyful. But the principle of "wholeness" for humans is a mystery in that it is never fully achieved. Perhaps for ontological reasons, there is always another pain, hurt, or feeling of incompleteness that needs healing. There may even be a natural developmental order of incompletions to complete, so growing may proceed from one level or phase of wholeness to another, though the course of healing is very similar within each phase. But the human, as a very complicated system of sub-systems, is filled with many concurrent hurts, inadequacies, and incompletions, each with its own long history and intensity of pain or degree of incompleteness. Furthermore, healing one hurt or completing one phase may depend upon healing or completing some other hurt or phase. So many different healings may be occurring simultaneously, though it is the most painful that usually captures consciousness, sometimes obsessively so. Finally, healing, just like growing, can cease, become blocked or avoided at any time within the healing sequence or after the completion of a phase. We may be left with the illusion of recovery or wholeness. We may feel cured, but not be healed.

Psychic healing has its own natural sequence initiated by a hurt.

For me, healing had to begin by recovering my body's healthy functioning, the first phase of the journey my cancer had set me on. The hurt to my body turned me deeply inward, absorbed all my energy, accentuated my self-centeredness, forced me to become excessively aware of how unpredictable and out of control my body had become, particularly of its urinating and defecating. A measure of my healing was the progressive freeing of energy from concern for my body to become available for connecting with and becoming concerned about others and about my work. My inner physician, now assuming more and more direction of my healing, insisted that I alter my former way of life to create a more healthy and stable self, less susceptible to future disease and trauma. Not until I was tested would I know how healthily resilient I had become to new stress. Dismayingly, the escape of the cancer into the prostate's capsule precipitated a damned early test, but eventually I was able to bounce back.

The result of healing is transcendence.

As I gained increasing control of my body, I became freed to move to the next phase of reforming my sexual self. My body had become more reliable, its functions more habitual and automatic. The long-term effect of these trying months was to release large amounts of energy from my preoccupation with my body to become available for other healing. I now had a more detached perspective of my urinary trials and could smile, even laugh, about the bottles placed in strategic places around the house and about the leftover diapers I still kept in my closet. Transcendence made me feel stronger, more confident in my ability to confront whatever future illnesses, including cancer's recurrence, I might have to endure. The same effects occurred after completing other phases of my healing; they were signals that I had completed each phase.

A natural developmental order of incompletions to complete.

The course of my healing's phases mysteriously seemed to recapitulate my earlier development. The first phase completed the mastery of my body, when I had moved from my early helplessness and emerging self-consciousness toward the firm control of my bodily functions. Then, at a more complex level, I seemed to relive the phase of shaping my sexual identity. I repeated and reexperienced healing's natural pattern as I mourned the loss of the most visible and prized witness of my maleness. After turning deeply inward to rediscover autoerotically my body's sexual responsiveness, I began to turn outward to reconnect through memory with my adolescent peers. Miraculously, I met a young man through whom I completed some unfulfilled youthful needs and rediscovered my full orgasmic potential. I was now ready to extend my refound sexual potential to Maryjane by finding new ways to integrate it with my love for her. But my inner physician intervened.

As a "system," a human has many concurrent incompletions.

By this time I had learned that the course of psychic healing was far from being a simple linear movement to an argument's conclusion, my preferred approach to a problem. Healing was not to be understood by a course in logical argument! While I was absorbed by one phase, my busy inner physician had been working on other phases concurrently. Hints of his labor frequently occurred, alerting me to trials to come; one such hint was his clever ploy of having me associate to "cancer" after associating to "cock," months before I was ready to feel the disturbing meanings that cancer was provoking on a less conscious level.

Completing one phase may depend upon healing's course in other phases.

I was unable to complete my sexual incompleteness with Maryjane, for my inner physician believed that I had to mourn my own death before I could find a new way by which to love Maryjane more completely. By mourning the most visible sign of having had cancer, the death of Old Faithful, he had been wisely preparing me for the next and more obscure phase of my healing, accepting dying.

So again I reluctantly traveled the familiar healing route to understand cancer's meaning. My depression drew me very far inward; I did not understand myself for months. As I began to accept my own losses, I turned to struggle with what my dying might mean to others and what my relation would now be with them. But in a very painfully perverse and complicated way, I had to learn how to accept the most central of Death's demands: give up not just my cock, which had connected me to others in the past, but also, and more painfully, the immature parts of my emotional connections to those whom I loved. Only after traveling this path would I be prepared to affirm what life was to mean for me in the future and what my relation with Maryjane was to be as a consequence. Because I have not yet been tested by Death again, I do not know if I have really transcended it. My current effort to form a sounder and more realistic view that could sustain me in the years ahead when meeting Death and its emissary, aging, therefore may not be fully integrative. This phase remains incomplete.

The most painful captures consciousness, sometimes obsessively so.

Mourning the death of Old Faithful was the principal route to my self-healing. My cock's centrality to my identity made its death the most palpably painful of my losses. But, as my inner physician told me, my obsession with my impotence had been "carried to a dogma." I had lost perspective.

Healing could cease, be blocked or avoided.

If I had not had such a determined and perceptive inner physician guiding me, I might well have settled for Dr. Paul's verdict that I had been "cured" of cancer. After regaining my physical health, I could have returned to my former way of life, ignoring the meanings of impotence and of cancer. Avoiding impotence's threat to my view of myself and my deepest feelings about my own maleness could have left me and my relationship with Maryjane vulnerable to future frustration, bitterness, resentment, maybe even physical symptoms. Ignoring cancer's threat to my life could have left me very vulnerable, not only to its recurrence but also to aging and any other intimation of death.

Meditations on maleness

What did my associations to "cock" tell me I could now affirm about my maleness? I had been shocked by my responses of "natural law" and "God" and puzzled why I had said "maleness" after "God." Logically, I should have thought of "maleness" as my first response to "cock." Just chance? Not likely. My trial work has taught me to observe witnesses carefully for just such coincidental subtleties that might suggest hidden meanings and motives.

My first two revelations told me that my cock stood for the life-force, a natural, biologically given, vibrant will that actively sought to connect, combine, and create deepening ties with others. Maryjane said I would like Freud's concept of Eros, a drive to create erotic ties with others. I did, for I have long felt Eros to be the underground stream suffused through much of my life.

What were the signs of my life-force? Very high energy and productivity that came from constitutionally high stamina; disciplined channeling of energy for sustained periods; a variety of talents demanding to be used; a sensitive autonomic nervous system that made me responsive, occasionally too much so; persistent sexual fantasies and intense desires; enjoyment of my sensuality; enthusiasm; the capacity to feel passionately; an abiding curiosity and restless need to explore, move, and create, which had never left me bored; plans and more plans; projects and more projects; this book. I was at the frontier of ideas in my field, future-oriented, willing to try new technology. I was one of the first lawyers to use computers, though my partners were skeptical about their usefulness to the firm. I left my firm because it was becoming full of "dead" people who stifled my growth. I gravitate toward people who are alive, vital, interesting, and exciting, avoiding if I can the sodden and dull who have little erotic spark or color. I am open to interpersonal risk and adventure. My life force probably also shows itself in my persistent denial of death and resistance to thinking about it, as well as in my being possessed by an inner physician who demands that I grow and gives me access to deeper sources of energy, power, and insight than I can reach alone.

Could I understand more deeply what this life-force might be by asking what mutes its force, that is, what is dying?

Dying is closing oneself off to life's energy, interest, vitality. Dying is blocking, suppressing, numbing, dampening, repressing, hiding, constricting, contracting, impairing, reducing sexual desire and other desires as well. Dying is pessimism, hopelessness, declining expectations, but also guilt, recriminations, lingering hostilities. Dying is the diminution of *joie de vivre*, enthusiasm, excitement, and responsiveness. Dying is severing ties to the world; losing friends and loved ones; diminishing sight, hearing, touch—all of those bodily sensitivities that heighten contact with the non-self. It is self-centeredness. Dying can also involve great efficiency and orderliness, which represent too-intense channeling of the self at the expense of emotional spontaneity, playfulness, responsiveness— the routes to systemic wholeness. It means not stretching, expanding, adventuring, risking, discovering, fulfilling. Dying is retarding, slowing, or stopping growth. A bit of dying occurs every time we ignore a potential to be realized, neglect a talent, fail to reach out to a person who attracts us. So although living is dying, because we cannot explore all of our potentialities, it is our life-force's strength that postpones death's claims.

What had God meant to me by the time of this nine-month perspective? My practical, down-to-earth, skeptical, rational mind had never really been bothered by the question of God. But obviously, my inner physician had been. How do I know? Many little signs during my healing. Upon leaving the firm and relocating to a smaller office in my home, I had to discard a large number of books not related to my work. When finished, I was startled to see that I had unconsciously placed my books about religion next to the sexual fiction on the adjacent shelf.

Why did I put sex next to religion? I think there is a real meaningful connection here. Sex has always caused problems for religions. Some religions so revere life-giving cocks that they create monuments to and ceremonial celebrations about them. Others repudiate any ideas of a cock. I think of the celibate priests, enjoined from all sexual temptation and pleasure. Is there spiritual wisdom in that proscription? What is more earthy, distracting, and complicating than an erection's tingling, exciting, vibrating elevation? What impels action into the world as vigorously or the urge to "plough" fields as deeply? Until this core meaning of maleness is overcome, repressed, put aside, transcended, I suppose a man cannot really fully submit to the will of God. An erection is always potentially willful, as I know, and can get in God's way. Maybe that is why priests who have devoted themselves to snuffing out their sexuality in the service of God do not seem to me to be very masculine, passionate, or sexual. Am I having a real struggle with God? If so, my cock is at the core of it.

Another sign that I was being troubled by God was my rejection of Christ as a model for my life.

We sang hymns this morning that exhorted us to become like Jesus. One had words like, "Purify me of the passion of desire so I may have a more calm inward spirit." During the baptism of an infant that followed, we responded with "Yes, yes, lord, I do" and "I agree" to the minister's statements about resisting or giving up temptations of the flesh.

Why did I sing those hymns and respond, "I agree"? I don't want to be like Jesus. I have no aspirations to be a saint. Christianity, as I experience it, too severely denies the body, which is God's temple of the spirit, sensuous responsiveness, sexual passion, and eroticism. Dying to Christ is dying to one's own body. A part of my body has died as a result of my surgical baptism, and I don't like the result one bit. My sexual desires are not sinful. I enjoy being tempted and seduced, as well as tempting and seducing. Sex is tumult and disturbs my inward calm spirit. Marvelous! Anger, envy, and greed don't motivate or inspire me. It is the erotic that intrudes, complicates, provokes ups and downs, makes me feel alive. I cannot see Jesus as an intensely sexual or passionate person. Thirty is an awfully young age to have repressed or transcended the desires of the flesh. No, I have no desire to be a monk. I could never see myself as a saint. Nor could anyone else who knows me.

Finally, after hearing a sermon on God and evil, I again rejected traditional religious views of my world.

Did God create evil? If He created the world, why is there so much evil? Is it God's will that we are on the verge of blowing ourselves up? Is cancer God's way of punishing me for trespassing against my nature? These questions drearily pass me by. I am a thoroughgoing naturalist. I have not found accepted religious beliefs helpful to me on my journey through cancer. Is not being able to accept and submit to some authority other than my own experience just another example of my pride? If I were closer to death than I am now, would I feel differently?

No wonder I was shocked at my impetuous associations of "natural law" and "God" to "cock." Damn! Why?

Cocks and natural law.

Penises and vaginas are biological givens and their meanings follow natural laws of male and female development whose centuries-long mysteries, so Maryjane tells me, researchers are just beginning to understand. My experience as a male is very unlike her experience as a female, and vice versa. Someday a woman may write a book about the meanings of her vagina to help clarify where our experiences may be more similar than I now think. Differences between the male experience and the female experience far transcend only genital-generated differences in attitudes, values, and views of our masculinity and femininity. Neurological research suggests the rate and type of brain development differ for men and women, and despite apparent dispute, psychological studies show modal male and female differences that seem to match those that neurohormonal research is suggesting. Some even suggest that because each of us has a male and a female brain, we all contain the potentialities of the opposite sex, though typically the brain appropriate to our gender becomes more differentiated.[1] Our maleness or femaleness may be more subtly suffused throughout our system than we now know.

For example, males tend to be much more analytically focused and single-minded, logically plunging ahead to the bottom line, frequently ignoring more contextual clues. Females, however, tend to note many more seemingly "irrelevant" cues, seek to grasp contexts, think more holistically and systemically, and therefore are more able to deal with complexities, particularly interpersonal and emotional ones, which makes women seem more intuitive and perceptive.

Our sexual differences may be similarly organized. My sexuality is much more focused than is Maryjane's. My penis was the gathering place for all kinds of vague and specific erotic feelings. When it defied gravity, it became a very visible agent of my desire, concentrated and absorbed my consciousness, and so created all kinds of problems for me. Affirmation of my cock "into a dogma" was a predictable outcome of my more analytic, focused male mind. A vagina may not create the same meanings. A woman's erotic feelings are more diffused, apparently not so concentrated, certainly not so visible, and they become more blended, I think, with a much more rich complex of interpersonal emotions. A woman's predictable monthly period may have very different emotional meanings than a man's unpredictable daily erections have. Losing an erection may have more disruptive effects on a man than, for instance, a hysterectomy may have on a woman.

Cocks and God.

But what does God have to do with my cock, which is God's handiwork and whose meanings follow God's natural law? For me, my cock was the life-force. Surely the belief in God as creator is the most embracing of life-forces as well. My cock is God? At the very least that is considered blasphemy, the epitome of hubris, which was my first response to "cock." That was also my pathology, as my associations to "cancer" subsequently demonstrated. Once I had mourned and transcended Old Faithful, I began to see that God was the given organizing spirit and principle of wholeness for which my inner physician had been the agent.

Then, nine months to the day after he had begun revealing these insights, my inner physician revealed who he was, startling me with a cascade of all of the following answers to my mysteries.

I should have known who he was, but I had been blinded by my male mode of knowing. He was my feminine voice. More accurately, she was my feminine voice. What Maryjane said Jung called anima. She was my latent, subtly intuitive, perceptive, holistically unconscious self, more deeply in touch with my system's history and needs than was my more consciously focused self. She was my personal voice of God's systemic principle of wholeness, reminding me of inner distortions, sensing the healing direction I needed to travel, preparing me for transcendence. She was not God; she was my contra side. My path to wholeness led by way of accepting and integrating her strengths and perspectives into my more typically male mode of being. She pointed the way to salvation, reconcilation with the principle of God..

My inner physician also told me in her last creative moments why I had been able to follow her leads; why I'd been so willing to trust and submit to her guidance, follow her into very painful unconscious memories and desires, faithfully use my talking book to sensitize and articulate my intuitions and perceptions and to learn how to think more intuitively and systemically. By keeping open the potential of an expanding wholeness, the intuitive could become integrated with the more rational and logical. Maryjane had been my inner physician's supportive, visible representation.

Cocks and natural law, God, maleness.

Completing the mourning of my oldest and most intimate companion allowed me to transcend his former, largely unknown, hold on my deepest feelings of who I was. I found I could be a whole person without an erection, a psychically healthy male with only a penis. My life-force had been diminished somewhat: I was less responsive and spontaneous; channels for its expression had been reduced; I felt persistent regret and nostalgia when imagining my former cock, and experienced a daily reminder that I had cancer every time I saw or touched my limp penis. But my fear that the muting of my erotic voice might erode my imaginative creativity proved to be groundless, particularly as the voice of my inner physician became increasingly mine, so giving me access to my more intuitive and systemic modes of thinking.

I have come to this understanding of my associations. Accepting and fulfilling the needs and meanings of maleness as represented by an erect penis is part of a natural law for developing wholeness. The cock is a principal instrument for a man to affirm and celebrate the life-force. But maleness remains only self-indulgence, narcissism, and power if not integrated into a larger wholeness that brings into some harmonious unity the evolving contrasts and seeming paradoxes of our being. Maleness, symbolized by my cock's meanings, is my natural organizing focus, my way through which I am to reach and witness God. That is why "maleness" followed rather than preceded "God" in my associations. Since each additional step along the way to wholeness transcends the previous one and releases energy, the test of my evolving wholeness is the amount of energy I have for joyfully celebrating God.

Has not my pride now just been cleverly hidden under the cloak of a narcissistic view of God? I don't think so. For the natural law of human growth and healing and the directional movement of the life-force suggest that God's principle of wholeness applies not just to my skin-contained system but reaches out, embraces, intertwines with others, creating ever-larger self/other systems: friends, spouses, families, communities, regions, nations, our planet, the universe—with which we may feel a mystical unity. Each transcendence frees us of a little more of our narcissism. We then truly become pure instruments of the life-force.

Meditation on mysteries

The abiding mystery that shadowed every step along my route to healing was, "What was the meaning of that cancer"? What did "Death, nuclear destruction, humility, fall, fall of man, 'punishment,' day of judgment" tell me about cancer?

Only after I had worked my way through my depression, accepted my losses, and stumbled upon how I was to say goodbye to Maryjane, did my inner physician's purpose become clearer. She was telling me that the meanings of "cancer" were mine; they came from deep inside me and no one else. I had to accept emotionally that I'd had cancer, that the coming "day of judgment," "nuclear destruction," and "Death" were *my* day of judgment, the ending of *my* personal world and *my* path. Transcendence would not be found by following any other path.

The way to understanding my meanings opened when I asked another seemingly trivial question: Why did my physician have me associate first to "cock" and then to "cancer," when logically it was the cancer that had caused all of my problems with my dead penis? How do the meanings of my erection illuminate the meanings of my cancer?

The cancer occurred in my prostate, a sub-system of larger systems, eventually of me as a person-system. I must therefore seek cancer's meaning for me systemically—I have learned that from my inner physician.

Biologically, my cancer resulted from some disruption of my biochemical equilibrium that my immune system was unable to heal. Why this occurred remains a mystery, though dietary and emotional stress that impaired my body's resilience to fight off the cancer were probably contributory. My naturalist's mind rejected Freud's answer of an innately given death-wish actively goading me to die. Yes, I am genetically programmed to die, given that I have only so many cell divisions ahead of me. And yes, cancer is a *biologically* active death-force, but not a *natural* one, for it is not one of God's universal natural laws.

Psychologically, I had very early in my healing interpreted cancer to mean that my way of living had become so distorted that my body had rebelled. I was living to excess: I was not coping well with large amounts of intense emotional conflict; my many rich accumulating experiences were not well digested and needed interpretation; I was too externalized in the lives of my clients; my life was too closely scheduled and focused to allow time for listening to my inner voices.

Socio-culturally, as an American male I had created a way of life that channeled my maleness very effectively into culturally accepted and valued forms of analytical and logical power. Again, as an American male I valued disciplined self-control, a strong will, emotional self-sufficiency, independence, and high achievement. My inner physician had shown me that each of these values had been hidden in the emotional meanings of erections, and perhaps even found their genesis or at least support there. Impotence showed me just how deeply male I was. The key to understanding how my erection illuminates the meaning of cancer came from my most immediate response to the word "cock": hubris, which is overweening arrogance. My proud erection was so powerful that it could defy a natural physical law like gravity; I could indulge in its urgings for my own pleasure. The result was that I loved my cock, my maleness, myself more than I did God, which is the essence of narcissism, my ultimate hubris. No wonder I had so valued my male strengths like logical analysis and self-control and was so devastated by losing my cocky cock! My pride in my cock, in my maleness, blocked my continuing growth into a healthier wholeness that might have integrated the contra-sexual, the voice of my feminine inner physician.

The meaning of cancer, from this socio-cultural perspective, is that my male hubris impaired the health of my system by blocking its continued growth. Cancer was the "punishment" (Had I put it in quotes for violating a systemic, rather than a legal, principle?) that had resulted in the fall of my cock and impotence.

Historically, I may be a voice of every man, certainly of western man. Some sections of my path were not singular or singularly American. My associations with cancer may have tapped a deeper commonality of males' historical experience. Maryjane says Jung might interpret my cancer as the result of being possessed by a universally shared maleness/ power archetype that can produce pathology, particularly in males like me who overvalue logical reason at the expense of our more primitive mythological unconscious.

My hubris as a modern man is that I have arrogated to myself ultimate power to both destroy and create. Nuclear destruction and cancer are the two most feared scourges of our time. Using my male analytic and quantitative brain, I have secured control over ultimate destructive power. Cancer has become the scourge it is because of my scientific and technological power to create new chemicals and so to alter my planetary environment and atmosphere in ways that are killing me. I am even now on the verge of controlling the power to create life and thus to alter the course of my own evolution into greater realms of systemic complexity and wholeness through genetic engineering. The male principle is elevating me to the supreme height of narcissistic power. How far is my fall to be? Cancer tells me how fragilely unwhole my male power has made my world, myself, and every other person.

Religiously, I am every person since Adam and Eve from whom the themes of pride, temptation, self-indulgence, fall from God's grace, day of judgment, and "punishment" have been inherited. They so silently programmed my own personal story I was not aware of them until my inner physician revealed herself. Through them I have learned that my journey is that of every person. Cancer is alienation from God. Healing is the way back to the Garden.

Given how much I am under the control of hubris, I squirm to suggest that some parts of my journey may be every person's. But by accepting my cancer as a universally shared metaphor for the deadly illness our civilization faces and for the existential sickness of all of our cóllective souls, I am helped to transcend the immediacy of my personal hurt. Perhaps as I feel that collective identification more deeply, I will be able to abandon my narcissism to follow the path of humility and submit my will to God's.

12
A Golden Resurrection

For two more months my trial continued before the technological trans-formation of my limp penis into a more contemporary cock. My physician had gotten the time he had wanted to lead me further into the meaning of dying and beyond the biological and psychological meanings I had earlier discovered about my cancer. Failure to accept cancer as my own and so not begin to transcend its meanings might increase the risk of future illness. I needed to grow into a more embracing and healthier wholeness that would moderate my narcissism. Otherwise, my new technologically immortal cock could become my pride's instrument to continued defiance of God as well as to my denial of the natural law that the erections of mortal males must eventually subside and fall.

My devious inner physician had a more subtle reason for waiting those two months to decide about the implant. She apparently felt my decision to resort to technology had to be tested, and designed some cleverly provocative tests of my resolve.

As I meditated more deeply about my maleness and cancer, I became troubled by some meanings of my technological salvation. Shouldn't real transcendence of my impotence mean not needing or desiring an artificial cock? I began to doubt my resolve.

Yes, my technological solution solves the historic fear of all males that we may not be able to perform. Those transitory episodes of impotence and consequent moments of uncertainty, embarrassment and shame would be eternally banished from my life. My cock would never again be humbled. A technological miracle! An immortal erection! But form with no spirit? A pen with no ink? A plastic solution that is an illusion?

Walt Disney showed the great power that technological illusion has. Though we knowingly pay $18 to enter into his illusory world, we still can be frightened by the ghost that jumps out at us in his haunted house. But afterward, we know we have participated in an illusion, and we laugh.

With my technological cock, I can create the illusion of panting desire. I will have the power to manipulate the desire of others by sending messages I may not feel. Maryjane will never know how I am really feeling. My body will be able to lie. Some women have been upset by penile implants for this reason. Technology will give me the power to deceive and so control the most intimate feelings of others. I could laugh; they won't.

I risk violating my human authenticity in connecting with another with such technological power.

But then I thought of other technological wonders: trifocals that enable me to read the fine print in books, gold fillings that enable me to still enjoy biting and chewing, the hearing aid I may soon need that will enable me to keep in contact with others. My meditation ended with, "So symbolically, when I am replaced by mechanical-plastic parts, like a permanent erection, essentially eternal life, what is life's meaning to be then?"

Verses from three psalms helped me to subdue my doubts and affirm my technological cock's potential goodness:

What is man, that thou art mindful of him? and the son of man, that thou visitest him? For thou hast made him a little lower than the angels, and hast crowned him with glory and honour (Psalm 8:4,5).

I will praise thee; for I am fearfully and wonderfully made: marvelous are thy works; and that my soul knoweth right well (Psalm 139:14).

Thou wilt shew me the path of life. In thy presence is fulness of joy; at thy right hand there are pleasures for evermore (Psalm 16:11).

The Psalmist is not singing a paean to our pride or narcissism; he is affirming how "fearfully and wonderfully" we are made, almost like angels, in the image of God, and that glory, honor, fullness of joy, and pleasures follow when we walk the path that leads to greater wholeness.

My conclusion? My path to wholeness was not to deny but to affirm how fearfully and wonderfully I have been made as a male. A resurrected cock could celebrate my maleness and nurture the life-force, *if* it were integrated with a more healthy embracing wholeness.

Had I only cleverly used the Psalmist's words to justify continuing self-indulgence and narcissism? I didn't know, since I had not yet gotten my new cock to test its effects. But I did feel I was at a different level of wholeness by now. I felt I had transcended Old Faithful's death and former centrality to myself. I had begun to become more aware of my pride and how it may have led to my illness. So I was more mindful that I was "a little lower than the angels." After all, "humility" had been one of my associations to "cancer," though I have yet to learn how to take that path.

Along technology's path to wholeness

I planned to celebrate the anniversary of my impotence by making an appointment to get my erection back. I did not make the appointment. My inner physician intervened again. The night before, I experienced what I called the first of numerous "perverse miracles." I awoke in the middle of the night with a pain in my penis. It felt hard like a bone. Sleepily, I touched it. The bone disappeared. The same sensation the next two nights. Maryjane's smirk said, "I told you so." I was bewildered. The urologists were certain I was permanently impotent. I might have a partial erection but unless it persisted for more than twenty minutes, I probably could never have intercourse with it.

Was I hallucinating? I needed evidence. Every night for weeks I pasted a ring of postage stamps around my limp penis to see if the ring was torn the next morning. What joy when I discovered it was. What despair when it wasn't. Still, this was really not evidence. I would only believe my eyes. So I tried to keep one eye open during the night to catch a look before it started to disappear. Of course, I was not successful since spontaneous nighttime erections occur only in deepest sleep. Would Maryjane stay awake and monitor Old Faithful's resurrection during the night? Her grimace told me that idea was not going to work. Meanwhile, believing that my experimental nerve regeneration treatments were beginning to have an effect, I redoubled their application. After beginning to feel more tingling, warmth and movement in my penis, I wrote, "I do not feel so dead there, but then again, how much of this is a wishful reaction I don't know. So to be conservative, I still am not raising my hopes too much."

But what to do? I felt confused, uncertain. I thought I had finished mourning my cock. I was eagerly excited about getting my new one and felt like I did when I had anticipated shopping for my first car. I also was very curious to discover what effects it would have on me and my relationship with Maryjane. She again suggested that I wait a year. Another year without sex when I didn't know how many more years I really had left to enjoy it? What would another year do to our relationship? To my sexual desire for her? The depth of my despondency on the mornings the ring of stamps remained intact told me how severely my inner physician was testing my resolve.

After a month of this frustrating trial, I had no lingering doubts. It was time to go ahead with the implant operation, which I would have after my visit to England to see my son. Upon my return home, I wrote:

In a week I resort to technology to deny death, which may not be the way to say it accurately. As a result of my visit with Pete and my discovery of how to say goodbye to Maryjane, I feel ready to move on. I no longer feel depressed. I feel I have finally accepted my impotence. My nightly wishful erections have disappeared. I can continue to have orgasms by masturbating. Maryjane is content with our existing nonsexual relationship. I could become so, if I had another, more sexual relationship. The implant will activate the more adventurous, playful, erotic, expressive, exciting side of me; it will provide more opportunities for connecting with others and hopefully with Maryjane. So I look forward to the process and to the end result, despite the complications it may bring. Eros will still triumph—for a while.

Maryjane's contentment with her "sexual" (actually just playful hugs and kisses), but my nonsexual, fulfillment had sparked occasional irritability, even spasmodic resentment, those five months:

Increasingly, I feel my penis has become irrelevant to her life and values, and that she not only views it as useless but also possibly as a hindrance to her own future happiness. I get too many cues—not ones of commission but ones of omission—that she may actually be becoming averse to it. She has reached out only once, and very tentatively at that, to touch it. I sense almost a feeling of relief that I am impotent, not just because she may feel sex to be more a drain than a fulfillment, but also because she may feel impotence will keep me emotionally tethered to home. She is very Puritanical and may not want me to have the sexual enjoyment she herself doesn't desire. These feelings are very real to me after 15 months of no sex. I hope I am misreading her feelings. Time will tell.

So typically male! It was some, though not much, comfort to then read Hite's sex survey results:

. . . the biggest complaint of men with heterosexual experience was that women didn't touch them enough . . . they didn't seem interested or they lacked the know-how. . . .[1] When asked what they would like to change about sex, the most common answer by far was: no change, just more. This complaint was . . . more pronounced in men in longer marriages, but in fact, throughout all the answers to all the questions, from men of every age and situation—married, single, or living with a woman—this was the complaint heard most frequently: I want more sex than she does. I never get enough sex.[2]

Eagerly expectant, I entered a different hospital where my new urologist practiced. I had chosen him since he was an expert on the inflatable type of prosthesis.

Troubled that my operation was my decision only, and by Maryjane's distance, I wrote the following, between routine visits from nurses, the anesthesiologist, dietician, cardiologist, ward physician, residents, and a trip to the x-ray department:

Is this folly? I may be getting a very expensive toy, not just in terms of its exorbitant cost, but also in terms of risk to my life now and in the future if it needs repair. What if there is an infection? But more importantly, I risk discovering that my sexual responsiveness to Maryjane may diminish if after the operation I find she is not responsive. I told her my feelings: I understood and accepted the primacy of her professional work over our sexual relations; I had felt some lessening of the emotional richness of our relationship during the past few sexless months; I was getting the implant primarily for me and would not make demands of her, but I wanted to be able to love her in my special ways if ever she wanted me to. I felt good about my decision and looked forward to the operation.

Maryjane again went with me to the operating room. Her strained face and forced smile brought back earlier memories of uncertainty and fear. But I felt good, joked with the residents, insisted on a spinal so I could watch the proceedings, but then fainted from the pain of the anesthetic needle. The operation and postoperative recovery went flawlessly. I reacted like an old hand. Four-hundred-and-seventeen days after losing Old Faithful, I awkwardly walked out of the hospital with his heir hanging heavy between my legs.

For those who ever plan to trade in their original cock for another: What was it like to get a new model?

My penis is huge. It is swollen, very purplish from the blood that has engorged it. It is very sore. I have problems with such a large, sore penis, for it gets in the way of walking and sitting. I feel it swing back and forth when I walk; it hangs heavily. I can feel the walnut-sized pump in my right scrotum, and the ring around the top, which, when squeezed, will deflate my erection; the extension of the cylinders down into the base of the penis; the tubes from my scrotum up into my groin. All of this gadgetry makes my penis stiff. But it is a good feeling to feel such a huge thing lying along my leg. It's 4½ inches long, 5¾ inches in girth at the base.

My recovery sped along very rapidly, according to my remote and detached urologist. I was sore but did not experience the severe, prolonged pain I had been warned about. I never had to take the prescribed narcotics. Could it be a sign of my wholeness that I was feeling pain as only soreness?

A week later, I said:

I seem to have gotten more than I bargained for—or anticipated! And while I am pleased with my huge penis, it causes complications. Maryjane's smiles of "I told you so" don't contain much sympathy but she has been very caring. My resurrected penis is a real handful. It juts out at about a 60 degree angle. Since it doesn't droop or curve into my scrotum, I have trouble keeping it in my jockey shorts or getting it out to urinate. I certainly can no longer complain about not being fully packed; its girth is really impressive. It is so big, it no longer has any wrinkles. It looks youthful again. I wonder where the skin is going to come from when it becomes erect. But it is very tender and sore to the touch. When I sit down, I sit on its tip, which is very sore. They got the cylinders into my glans by pushing needles through the tip and pulling the cylinders behind them.

My new penis has a very special appeal to me. I feel very maternal about it, trying to take care of it, protect it, soothe it. Almost as if it is like a baby whom I wish to protect. Of one thing I do feel certain—I don't want to trade it back in for my old one.

As the swelling receded so did my penis's soreness. By fiddling with the pump, I could decrease its angle of inclination to a more manageable 35 degrees. Given its increasing flexibility, I could hide just enough of it to leave a slight, tempting bulge. After three months, the soreness had left. I was no longer aware of the pump and tubes. My cock had become mine.

A tarnished golden cock

Within a month of the operation, I got copies of the hospital's and surgeon's bills for Stubby, my nickname for Old Faithful's heir. Unbelievable. Despite my prior efforts to get realistic comparative estimates from three hospitals and urologists, the maximum being $10,000, Stubby's total cost was more than $15,000! Appalled, livid, furious, I called the hospital to demand a full accounting and advised the insurance company to do likewise. How could the total costs of my previous two more serious, life-threatening, and complicated operations, requiring extensive medical technology, two weeks of hospitalization, and much more intensive nursing and physician care, cost only $3,520 more than Stubby did? No rational explanation occurred to me. So I again concluded that it was sheer exploitation by the medical profession of an impotent middle-aged man's vanity and vulnerability.

My financial calculations about the cost of each orgasm had turned out to be about as reliable as the Defense Department's are for each missile blast! I figured that Stubby was a candidate for Fort Knox, being worth about 35 ounces of pure gold at the then-current London fixed price. I wouldn't have gotten him if I had known what his true cost was going to be.

Would I return Stubby if I could? No. Not because the value of technological cocks depreciates to zero once they are used, but because his effects on my emotional life and feelings about myself are worth many more ounces of gold than his current market value. Though the costs of his resurrection blemished my feelings about his rebirth, I have since become more good-humored and can even laugh about this tarnishing episode.

Fifty-percent fulfillment

I patiently waited 37 days for the first of three big anticipated moments. With high expectations, I watched as the doctor pumped and pumped to convert my penis into a cock. It painfully but firmly rose to a full rigid 90 degree "at attention" salute. A technological miracle had occurred 14 months after Old Faithful had died. But while bigger in girth when erect than Old Faithful was, it was also two inches shorter. I was crestfallen—it was only 4½ inches long! I hadn't been told that. I should have known. The advantage of the type of prosthesis I had selected was that its firmer cylinder walls meant it might hold up longer. Only now I realized that the trade-off was that my cock would not stretch when inflated.

The second big moment came that evening. I impatiently waited for Maryjane to turn into the driveway. As she did so, I hurriedly undressed, pumped up Stubby, tied a big red bow around him, and met her at the door beaming. She blushed. There was no blanket this time to teach him modesty. But it didn't matter, since he was too sore to use; I learned more about patience.

The third big moment came 15 days later, 446 days since Old Faithful succumbed to Dr. Paul's knife. Stubby seemed to be ready. I certainly was. Then I discovered Murphy's dismal law. If anything can go wrong, it will. Initially, I had enthusiastically pumped Stubby up so much that he yelled with pain when I unleashed him for action. Then, I found he was still very sensitive to pressure. But when he got a brand new slippery coat, he didn't feel anything. Next, I discovered that thousands of trials learning to thrust his predecessor had created an unconscious pattern of loving that was beyond Stubby's capability. He kept retreating too far. It took time to unlearn my physiologically ingrained habits, making me too self-conscious about how Stubby was doing. Even after trying all of the reputed Hindu positions of which we still were physically capable, I still had not recovered my orgasm with Maryjane, though I could by myself. As Stubby's tenderness subsided, I discovered he was much less sensitive to stimulation than his predecessor; he needed much more persistent and intense stimulation than our efforts were producing. Then I began to wonder if Stubby needed longer rest periods between his exertions. And on and on.

Was I undergoing another trial? Had I deluded myself about having completed earlier phases of my healing? Was I being "punished" for my pride in Stubby? Had all of that internal gadgetry become only a more intricate hiding place for my narcissism? At some very profound level of being, was I conflicted and guilty about my technological solution? Was I really defying natural law and God?

I was inclined to answer no to each question. My hunch was that my penis and I had been so mangled, violated, needled, and irritated from the two operations and their consequences that my cock had become desensitized and so required more violent and persistent physical stimulation and more novel and exciting psychic stimulation.

Why did I prefer this hunch? Simply because my feelings about this phase of my trial seemed to emerge more as transcendent than desperate reactions. I felt content that I was able now to love Maryjane again in my way and give her fulfillment. I had my answer to that nagging question, "How do I love you now?" And 50 percent was 1000 times better than zero, even though that 50 percent was not mine. My dilemma became our dilemma, bringing us much closer to as open and honest a sexual relationship as I could wish. Maryjane became much more playfully experimental and responsive than I had anticipated, and was now traveling the same road I was.

My own attitude and feelings about sex had changed from what they had been for the preceding 27 years of our married life. Now, not feeling desperate or defeated, I was able to joke about Stubby and my dilemma. I began to accept that sex might be evolving different meanings for me. I could be content about a relationship in which I could express my love for Maryjane, even though 100 percent mutual fulfillment might not come by my preferred ways. Maryjane said that she felt inadequate. I didn't think that she was; it was my problem now, not hers. We would create alternative ways if the conventional ones ultimately did not work out. I could not have accepted such views if my cock had remained so central to my sense of self. I would have been more serious, defensive, and worried.

A technological cock's effects

Stubby's arrival had numerous effects, some anticipated, some of the more important ones not anticipated. Sexual relations resumed. Whereas before it had been my ability to have an erection that had decided when we could have sex, now that Stubby could become fully primed in 12 seconds whenever we wanted him, sex became potentially more frequent. Greater honesty was required of us both about our needs and desires. And yes, I got more furtive stares from the men at the health club. And yes, one young man did casually tell me I had "a lot of muscle there," but added, to my irritation, "for an old man." Clearly, the path to humility was going to be a long and difficult one.

Because Stubby doesn't shrivel up and is much more firm and, well, stubby, I am more aware of his presence at all times. So Stubby remains more in mind. And despite what I had read, he is not a cold but quite a warm companion. On very cold days, though, his tip chills more readily.

I had not anticipated other important effects. Stubby has created the comforting illusion that I had never had cancer. For 446 days, my dead, thin, limp penis had been "a visible reminder of the fact that I don't have many more years to live." Some illusions are indeed benevolent and contribute to a more optimistic and healthier sense of self.

Stubby also told me I was no longer a sexual cripple. Even though I felt I had accepted and overcome my impotence, seeing and feeling its visible witness many times a day for 446 days had constantly reminded me of my handicap. Since my cock's resurrection, I have not once thought about parking in the A & P's empty spaces for the handicapped. I have transcended a deep narcissistic injury to my image of myself as a healthy, adequate male.

Though Stubby is more physically present than my former dead penis, I am not as absorbed with him. I had been growing away from such self-absorption prior to my cock's return, but Stubby gave me a big shove away from being as morbidly self-conscious about my dead penis as I had been, particularly around other nude males.

Another unanticipated and surprising effect was that Stubby turned out to be very erotically provocative, not because he could change his size, which he couldn't, but because of his prominent stubbiness; he is fuller, much firmer, almost semi-erect, because of all of his inner tubing. And I react with an erotic glow every time I see or touch him. Stubby has taught me that the desire men have for large cocks may stem in part from a semi-conscious feeling of being erotically aroused by seeing or feeling a large cock. It is an emotional reminder of a beginning erection. Anyway, I find I am more erotically primed now by Stubby. And being more primed has made me more accessible to other, less conscious, streams of feelings and ideas. Paradoxically, technology has made me feel a little more alive and lively.

Stubby has also required greater honesty about how I really feel and more self-restraint, which I have had trouble learning. My erotic life is more easily led now by my mind's fantasies than by my body's needs. The saying, "The spirit is willing but the flesh is weak" has a different meaning to me now. I can make my flesh, Stubby, more willing. I can create more easily now the illusion that I feel sexy. Whereas before, my cock would not only tell me when I was feeling sexy, it would also tell me when I wasn't. Now, I have no such bodily sentinel. So the temptation is to think I feel sexy and raise him up, only to find that I can't have an orgasm without great effort. Might the temptation to summon too frequently the technological illusion of sexual desire diminish genuine desire and mute orgasmic fulfillment?

Finally, now that my technological cock is no longer such a transparent mirror of my desire and not so central to my emotional identity, I find I am freer to be more humorous, playful, and expressive with my sexuality. I sometimes refer to Stubby as my "toy." On the one hand, such a feeling expresses transcendence over the glorified place my penis had held in my values; on the other, it reminds me of the dehumanizing effect that my technological illusion can have upon my sexual, and, eventually, interpersonal relationships.

Physically cured and psychically healed

The final entries in my talking book, beginning on the 463rd day after Dr. Paul's first telephone call:

> I feel very good about myself, the decisions I have made, how I have lived through the past year and a half, and where I am now. I feel much clearer inside. Despite its costs, I feel very good about getting my erection back. My pubic hairs are coming in and in a month or two, I will even appear normal. I have not been depressed for months, ever since working through my feelings about Pete and Maryjane. So all in all, it is an "up" time. It is good to feel so alive again.

> Day 466
> I haven't felt as light, effervescent, and responsive since before my illness. I now feel freer of myself than ever before.

> Day 481
> Today I have kept saying to myself how great I am feeling. My body is much more alive, as are my spirits. The cancer is far behind me now. My penis is much less sore. My days are full. With the one exception of not yet having an orgasm with Maryjane, I feel I am recovered.

> Day 514
> It has been more than a month since I have felt the need to reflect about my cancer. This is another sign of my increasing emotional

distance from it and my feeling that I have transcended its past and meanings, that my healing is about complete.

Day 532

I have little inner urge to reflect, which means many uncompleted tasks have been completed. And in one way, I do not feel any urgency to complete the orgasm with Maryjane, which will be great if it occurs. But I think more basically I have accepted where and what I am. I am beyond being upset by my stubby cock's petulance. He is enjoyable in his own right.I feel little pain or impetus to work on inner problems. I still mull over the last sign of the cancer, not yet having an orgasm with Maryjane. She has been very responsive and open to exploring and I appreciate her efforts to be helpful. Patience, Richard Handy, patience!

Day 547

I met my inner physician as the night's blackness began to recede. She revealed herself in a sparkling display of intuitive fireworks. Like a Roman candle she lit up my remaining mysteries, including her own being. I feel cleansed. What a beautiful day it is going to be.

Day 552

The healing of my impotence and cancer is now complete. I no longer feel the need for this talking book. I have learned about the art of healing myself and feel much more whole than I did before Dr. Paul's call. This journey is ended. I am ready for the next one.

Day 568

I will praise Thee. For I am a fearfully and wonderfully made male. In Thy presence is fullness of joy and pleasures for evermore.

Epilogue
Celebrating Maleness

Rereading this book since it was published eight years ago provoked five immediate impressions and then five questions.

My five impressions?

I had written out of much pain and emotional vulnerability whose intensity and depth I have not felt since.

I had turned inward more deeply than I had ever done before to get in touch with an inner insightful (dare I now write "wise") voice that I have not heard as clearly since.

The book openly described my experience as I lived it at the time and so should not now be revised, doctored, or sanitized to make it more acceptable to you—or to me and Maryjane.

My discovered meanings of my prostate cancer and former erections may have been ahead of their time; they may not now be, given that both are beginning to enter public consciousness as issues with which hundreds of thousands of men and their partners will have to come to terms in the immediate future.

And finally, not feeling defensive or rejecting but emotionally recognizing and accepting what I had written about the meaning of cancer and impotence told me I had transcended their past hold of me. I was now free to confront their longer-term effects, which my inner physician had begun to mumble about several months before my editor's request. I had heard my inner physician intimating that it was time to take stock of the effects of where I had been since 1988 and where I wanted to go the last part of my life. Actually, though much had changed, much had not.

And the five questions?

Has research since confirmed that we had made the right choices about my course of treatment?

How did I continue to cope with cancer's possible recurrence?

What does the explosion in research understanding of impotence suggest about my decision to replace Old Faithful by Stubby I and his heir, II?

What have been cancer's and impotence's lingering effects on my relationships?

What have been their lasting effects on my view of the mysteries of living: death, transcendence, and resurrection?

Did we make the right choices?

Yes. About surgery for the cancer. Do I have any regrets about surgery? No. That my cancer was more virulent than Dr. Paul first believed confirmed that Maryjane was right to insist that I get it out of my body immediately. Do I regret choosing surgery rather than only radiation therapy? No, not now. I fleetingly did when searching for my lost orgasms and erections. Why hadn't I selected a surgeon skilled in sparing the erectile nerves and so significantly reducing the risk of impotence by perhaps as much as 50 percent, though more recent research now suggests that the risk reduction may be by no more than 35 percent?[1] Discovering that I had a rapidly spreading cancer then made my question about a more skilled surgeon less pressing. Sparing my erectile nerves might have left part of a cancerous capsule.

Recent research suggests that our choice for surgery may have been right for me at the time.[2] Apparently other patients believe similarly. Surgery has increasingly become the treatment of choice, especially for younger men, now that improved surgical techniques do not automatically result in impotence;[3] between 1984 and 1990 there was a 5.75 increase in the rate of prostectomies.[4] Neurovascular preservation of erectile nerves is more successful in younger men who have early diagnosed cancer confined to the prostate, who have all of the nerves surgically spared, and who were vigorously potent preoperatively.[5] Also, death on the operating table has become much less frequent due to increased surgical control of blood loss,[6] and may become even less if experimental noninvasive treatments (e.g., laser[7] and laparoscopic methods[8]) eventually prove to be more beneficial. Also, evidence is accumulating that survival and disease-free rates for cancer confined to the prostate may be better than radiation therapy's, especially for younger men in their forties and fifties.[9] However, radiologists continue to question these comparative findings on the basis of studies that suggest no difference in long-term outcome for localized cancers.[10] The advent of more powerful targeted methods of radiation treatment such as three-dimensional radiotherapy[11] may enhance future survival rates as well as reduce the frequency of impotence.[12] Outpatient implantation of radioactive iodine seeds in the prostate has produced short-term results comparable to radical prostatectomies but its long-term survival rates and effects on potency are not yet known.[13] That we elected radiology to be our "insurance" policy in case of cancer's recurrence was also the right choice; surgery following radiology has been much less successful.[14]

I also do not regret our decision to have radiation therapy following surgery when told that cancer could have penetrated my prostate's capsule, which is subsequently found to have occurred in 25 percent to 50 percent of men undergoing surgery.[15] Dr. Paul was also right not to advise radiation therapy until I had fully recovered from the operation and I had become more continent.[16] Though postsurgery radiation may enhance the local control of cancer, the jury is still out that it contributes to disease-free long-term survival.[17] So it may have or may not have saved my life. I will never know. Whereas prostatic surgery that does not spare the neurovascular bundles governing erections almost guarantees impotence and increases the odds of urinary complications, radiotherapy aggravates bowel problems.[18] Whether due to aging or surgery, I urinate several times every night and every several hours; and I still suffer unexpected explosive defecations—embarrassingly once in the lobby of a four-star hotel. Ashamedly, I placated the maid who cleaned up the evidence with blushing apologies and a day's wages.

For cancer that has escaped the prostate's capsule, radiation and hormonal manipulation (whether by drugs or by removal of the testes) still remain the preferred recommended treatments rather than surgery. However, long-term survival rates for more than several years continue to be discouragingly low.[19]

Since the mid-eighties, several other treatment options have become more available, though their long-term survival and quality-of-life effects are as yet unknown. Combining drugs with surgical treatments is producing promising results. Administering drugs, such as flutamide, which block the production of testosterone several months prior to surgery apparently reduces the rate of cancerous penetration of the capsule and the volume of cancerous tumor; and it also possibly improves survival rates from the surgery.[20] However, the long-term biological effects and cancerous recurrence rates of such multitreatments are not yet known.

Another promising treatment is cryoablation, which involves freezing the prostatic cancer to destroy it. While not a new technique, the advent of ultrasound and other instrumentation improvements now enable more precise application of the cryoprobes, thus minimizing the destruction of surrounding noncancerous tissues. The reported reduction of metastases still must be confirmed by longer-term studies.[21]

In 1987, noninvasive laparoscopic procedures were first used to take out gall bladders. Three years later, pioneering urologists reported using such a procedure to stage the spread of cancer by dissecting the pelvic lymph nodes.[22] Such key-hole surgery involves the insertion of a miniature camera into the abdomen through a small incision to provide a two-dimensional picture on a television screen, enabling the surgeon to operate internally through two other holes without cutting open the abdominal wall. No longer need a man wake from an exploratory lymphadenectomy to see eighteen staples marching from his belly button to his pubic area! He will see only three small holes. And he will recover far more quickly from the operation. Since 1990, laparoscopy has been experimentally applied to many other organs; some adventurous urologists have used it to excise cancerous prostates but not without complications that have yet to be minimized.[23] Laparoscopy avoids the dangers of open abdominal surgery, its associated blood loss, and threat to mortality. However, training urologists to high-levels of competence in key-hole surgery, as well as reducing its greater costs due to longer operating times, may limit its widespread use[24] as hospitals and insurance companies seek to contain medical costs.

How to cope with cancer's possible recurrence

Dr. Paul warned that my cancer might recur five, ten, even fifteen years later, and he insisted that even after the fifth year I be checked twice a year for its metastasis to my bones and lymph glands. I was cured only provisionally. Several years of rectal and lymph examinations, occasional bone scans, and blood tests continued to prove negative for cancer.

In the meantime, new diagnostic technologies have become available that provide more accurate diagnoses of the odds that cancer may be present than digital rectal examinations suggest;[25] the latter examinations fail to discover as much as 40 percent of cancers subsequently found from biopsies.[26] Recent advances in ultrasound and imaging methods may detect cancer more effectively than rectal examinations, but some question their accuracy.[27] A more precise blood test measuring the amount of residual prostatic specific-antigen (PSA)—an indicator of possible prostate cancer—has since become the more widely used and extensively researched test.[28]

Agreement is emerging that combining these diagnostic methods results in detecting more cancers, possibly as much as "78 percent more organ-confined prostate cancers [with PSA] than would have been detected with rectal examination alone."[29] Though increased levels of PSA are regularly correlated with the increased odds of cancer's presence, biopsies still are necessary to confirm that cancer is actually present.[30] Other changes in the prostate, such as noncancerous infections or benign growths, can elevate PSA levels. PSA apparently more accurately predicts cancer's probability than does mammography for breast cancer.[31] PSA's availability, coincident with the arrival of the "baby-boomer" population into its forties and fifties, guarantees that many hundreds of thousands more men will be diagnosed with prostate cancer for years to come. Unless more effective treatments are discovered for the growing population of middle-aged men, an estimated 37 percent increase in deaths is likely to occur within five years.[32] Of most interest to me is that increasing PSA levels *after* treatment for cancer are especially diagnostic that therapy has failed, that residual cancer is present and growing, and that further treatment may be desirable.[33]

Since prostatic cancer's life-threatening potential arises from its possible migration to other parts of the body, identifying why metastases occur in some but not in other men is critical for improving diagnostic predictability and treatment efficacy. Recent research suggests that an anticancer gene exists that suppresses prostatic metastases and possibly other cancers, such as breast cancer and melanoma.[34] Since about 35 percent of men believed to have cancer localized to the prostate may have capsular involvement, other more accurate diagnostic methods, such as magnetic resonance imaging techniques, are being pursued.[35] A new diagnostic test, called RT-PCR, identifies special cells in the bloodstream that indicate prostatic cancer may have escaped the capsule. If its preliminary results can be confirmed, combining PSA and RT-PCR results will enable urologists to target treatments more effectively.[36]

Reassuringly, my PSA levels have remained low for the last four years. Despite the increasingly favorable omens that I am probably free of residual cancer, I have not abandoned efforts to forestall its recurrence. Given its long dormant time to recur and a character not built to do nothing in the face of the unknown, I have continued my campaign to stay cancer-free. But what more to do?

The critical unknown still remains: Why me? What caused my cancer? Patrick Walsh, who pioneered the identification of the nerve paths that control erections,[37] summarizes the possible causes, as of 1994, to be:[38] increasing age, altered hormonal environment, total fat consumption, *reduced* sunlight that may limit Vitamin D intake (hurrah for sunbathing—with discretion!), positive family genetic history,[39] and racial differences. Afro-Americans are more at risk for prostate cancer than Western European, Canadian, and American whites; Asians are less at risk, until they move to America and its high fat diet.[40] Smoking may contribute to prostatic cancer by suppressing the immune system's ability to combat it.[41]

Despite these hopeful new tests and a growing understanding of prostatic cancer's causes, the research to date still does not provide a better answer to why I got cancer than a high-fat diet, character traits, and stress. My initial promising preventive efforts to better regulate my diet continue to flounder because of my unreliable will-power. I cringed rereading page 82 to discover how far the tide of my high dietary resolutions had retreated. Gravies and whipped cream are just too addictive to overcome. The new Federal Drug and Food Administration (FDA) labels for the amount of saturated fat in my favorite foods are so depressing that if I were not on another campaign to still fit into my shrinking pants I would be unable to resist second helpings of either— or double first helpings!

Pete, more than Maryjane, who has resigned herself to my aversion to her barely cooked vegetables and rabbit food, still smirks about my addiction to meat and gravy. However, I do feel more virtuous nowadays: I actually have learned to enjoy mushy broccoli, cabbage, and spinach salads. I welcome the recent Harvard study[42] according to which the eating of ten servings of tomato sauce a week may reduce cancer's incidence by 45 percent! But ten servings? What next on this dietary see-saw?

My nemesis is my character. Frontal attacks to change it don't work over the long haul. I apparently value self-control so much because I don't have as much as I wish I had. Indirect efforts to change my character have been more successful—until recently.

My belief that stress and my ways of dealing with it precipitated the cancer by suppressing my immune system's ability to cope has now received some experimental support. Stress-reduction programs, such as progressive muscle-relaxation techniques and support groups, may increase natural killer-cell counts and reduce mortality.[43] So I have persisted to reduce stress and to consciously alter how I cope with it. I continue to follow my body's lead to seek that way of life which makes it feel more vibrantly alive and healthy.

The easiest stress to limit was that of nature's harsh winter weather and steamy sweaty summers. Leaving my law office and having the resources enabled me to move my office in the winter to my Mexican Puerto Vallarta time-share condo, where I feel much more at peace with my body and nature. There my fingers and feet never freeze, the tips of my fingers do not become painfully white, and clinging thermal underwear, two pairs of socks, and heavy sweaters are only irritating memories. Wearing only shorts all day wakens my body's feeling of freedom. The open doors of my balcony welcome the ocean's breezes that stroke my skin to make it feel more alive. The condo's large swimming pool invites daily swims and sunbathing. I then escape the hot sultry summer months that so depress me by going to our seacoast retreat. There I harmoniously live with nature's warm days and cool evenings; there I also abandon my rigorous consulting and writing schedules to live more serenely with the rising and setting sun and the tide's rhythms.

My body continues to demand daily, vigorous, physical stimulation. Exercising every morning every day for half an hour, climbing steps two at a time, swimming during the winter, gardening and working in my woods in the summer, hiking in the Philippines's Sierra Madre mountains and Luzon's rice-terraced countryside, swimming in the clear water of its coast during the fall and spring, and receiving too infrequent vigorous massages tell me what my body needs to feel alive.

My declining physical strength, stamina, and memory tell me I am aging. My occasionally uncontrollable and explosive bowel movements and incontinent dribbling when not consciously emptying my smaller bladder fully are enduring legacies of surgery and radiation which aging will continue to aggravate.[44] I continue to learn how to live with my body's increasing undependability and its consequent unpredictability—a lingering emotional threat to a man who has always valued self-control. Only hiking in the wilderness frees me from keeping a toilet's availability always close to awareness. I go to the toilet whenever near one; I sit on a plane's aisle seats to be able to get to the toilet in a hurry; I still carry an empty bottle in the car in case I get stuck in a traffic jam; I try not to drink much before going to bed.

I am now content that I have done all that I can to cope with nature's aggravating stress. My body tells me it feels good. Tom's annual physicals agree. But one aggravating stress persists: what to do with Stubby II.

Should I have replaced Old Faithful with Stubby I and then Stubby II?

I now am not sure. I have continued to regret Stubby's shorter stature and reduced sensitivity and firmness. What happened to Stubby was not unique. Fifty percent of men's postoperative penile implants are shorter, 36 percent to 65 percent less sensitive, and 11 percent to 25 percent less firm.[45] Despite such consequences, I have been satisfied with my new erection, as have the great majority of men studied. I would not want to live with my former, reclusive penis. Erections are too important to me and most men to quibble about their imperfections. For me, however, Old Faithful's Olympic standards remained too high (in memory) for Stubby to reach.

But the doctors were right. Stubby had to be replaced because of leakage in his connections. While lying prone on a Filipino masseuse's table, she unexpectedly clambered on my back to massage it with her feet! Her forceful pressure fractured Stubby's inner workings; he lost his backbone. As with Stubby's birth, I felt no postoperative pain after a more mechanically reliable Stubby II's difficult two-hour delivery. My urologist had never tried to free a deceased Stubby from his erectile tissue-embeddedness in a way to leave as much of his natural inner sponginess, or corpora cavernosum, as possible. I am proud of Stubby II's greater girth due to the insertion of larger cylinders. He continues to attract furtive, and what I want to believe are envious, glances from my health club's other swimmers.

Unfortunately, Stubby II inherited Stubby's stature; more unfortunately, he now has a wimpy cold tip and is even less sensitive to stimulation. He feels nothing when his cold tip is blanketed by a condom. Why? Certainly not because of reduced sexual desire. I am just as vitally sexual and desirous as I recall being when I first discovered Old Faithful's adolescent secret power. Stubby II continues to need two to three exercises a week. Though the operations have not diminished my sexual desire, they may for others, as prostatectomy had done, for example, for 12.7 percent of men in one study and as reported by sexual counselors based on interviews with men who seek their advice.[46] Nor have the operations limited my orgasmic capacity—as some urologists claim to have recently discovered.[47] Where have these urologists been all of these years? Preoccupied by the biological and oblivious to the emotional complications of cancer and sexuality?

My earlier explanation for Stubby II's physical need for more intense erotic stimulation still holds. The mangling of his forebear by four operations on his sensitive tip had damaged the sensory nerves: first the ureter and bladder were explored; then the tip was excised to insert the intrusive catheter that I frantically tugged and tugged to get out;[48] and finally much of the cavernous spongy insides was twice removed to insert the two implants' two cylinders by pulling them through his tip. Some men who have had several implants also report reduced penile sensitivity and reduced satisfaction with their erections.[49]

I also had not regretted Old Faithful's surgical replacement by Stubby until I reviewed the burgeoning research since the mid-eighties on sexual dysfunction and its treatment. I learned that my urologists had not fully informed me of inexpensive nonsurgical options available at the time to reclaim my erection. Because of financial self-interest? Dr. Paul wanted $3000 to replace Stubby I—for his estimated ninety minutes of operating time. I sought a cheaper urologist.

Sexuality and cancer

But first what do we now know about sexuality and cancer? And then what do we now know about the causes of impotence and its treatment? Leslie Schover's thoughtful critique of the research on sexual activity and cancer stakes out what is and is not yet known:[50]

- prostate cancer most likely is *not* associated with frequent prior sexual activity, which might increase testosterone, which in turn is believed to nourish prostatic cancer cells
- frequent posttreatment sexual activity probably does *not* increase the likelihood of cancer's recurrence
- urologists' estimates of the rate of recovery of potency after surgery, radiotherapy, or hormonal treatment for cancer are probably too high; their too narrow definition of potency fails to take into account erectile firmness, loss of sexual desire and penile sensitivity, and the quality of orgasms without the ejaculation of sperm through the penis if the seminal vesicles had been removed during a lymphadenectomy
- surgery that spares the erectile nerves is most effective in preserving erections in men under fifty, i.e., "68 percent had erections that allowed vaginal penetration,"[51] but not for men over seventy.
- radiology may create erectile problems in 25 percent instead of the frequently cited 50 percent of men, once pretreatment health and cancer severity are taken into account
- altering hormonal levels or removing the testes to treat metastasized cancer results for most men in the loss of sexual desire, failure in erectile ability, and reduced capacity for orgasm[52]

Schover's felicitous conclusion appeals to me: healthy young men who have had localized prostate cancer and are strongly motivated sexually—like me—may be able to have a fully satisfying sexual life after surgery or radiotherapy. Counseling to better understand one's sexuality, altering sexual habits and relationships, treating any residual depression that can inhibit sexual desire and potency, and remaining patient for the months necessary for physical recovery to occur following surgery, when combined with newer medical treatments for impotence, can ensure increased potency for most men.

Definitions. causes, and treatment of impotence

DEFINITIONS. What have researchers learned about impotence since the upsurge of interest in it this past decade? The critical issue is: what does "impotence" mean? In 1992 the National Institutes of Health (NIH) convened researchers who agreed that impotence defined as the "inability . . . to attain and maintain erection of the penis sufficient to permit satisfactory sexual intercourse . . . has often led to confusing and uninterpretable results in both clinical and basic science investigations."[53] "Erectile dysfunction" should be substituted for "impotence" as a more "precise term" to "signify an inability . . . to achieve an erect penis as part of the overall multifaceted process of male sexual function." This definition was then modified to refer to "inability to achieve or maintain an erection sufficient for satisfactory sexual performance."[54] More precise? Scarcely to my legalistic mind. Does "erect" mean a 45- or 60-degree angle or firm enough to masturbate though not necessarily firm enough to enter a vagina or anus? Does "multifaceted process of male sexual function" imply "adequacy" and include strength of libidinal desire and orgasmic response and frequent exercise (how many times a month)? And who defines what "satisfactory sexual performance" means? Does not such a definition ultimately depend upon a man's *subjective* feeling of "satisfaction"?

By the NIH definition, I have no "erectile dysfunction." I can make Stubby II rise any moment I wish to about a 90-degree angle; he guarantees erectile immortality, at least until he wears out. But by the definition of the largest random survey of male impotence, the Massachusetts Male Aging Study, reported in 1994,[55] I am moderately impotent. Taking into account men's self-defined degree of potency—"frequency of erectile difficulty during intercourse, lower monthly rates of sexual activity and erection, and lower satisfaction with sex life and partner"[56]—enabled the researchers to measure *degree* of subjectively rated impotence and to pursue its correlates.

By the NIH estimates, 10 to 20 million men and by the Massachusetts estimates, 52 percent of its random sample of forty to seventy men (or 18 million men) are impotent to some degree. Given the size of the estimates, it is almost irrelevant whether the actual number is 10, 18, or 30 million—except to marketing heads of drug companies. Clearly, millions of men have less than fulfilling sexual lives, the psychic effects of which have scarcely been studied by researchers, especially those biologically oriented ones, to whom only a small fraction of the millions go for assistance. Might not these researchers' special sample skew their perceptions about the causes of impotence?

Given the extent of self-defined impotence, I found it discouraging and shocking that few psychologists and mental health researchers had studied the emotional effects of impotence. Of the 926 articles on impotence published between 1986 and 1992, only 13 percent were classified as concerned with impotence's psychosocial aspects.[57] No wonder my search to come to terms with the meaning of my erections and their loss has been a lonely one.

CAUSES. Until the early eighties, impotence had been believed to be caused primarily by psychological conflicts, therefore not within the province of the urologists. The past decade has seen the pendulum swing to the opposite extreme. Now, some claim that 85 percent of men's impotence is caused by organic problems,[58] a highly debatable figure, given the lack of methodologically sound studies of a national sample of postpubertal males. Even the Massachusetts study of a nonclinical sample of forty- to seventy-year-old men found that of the 27 percent of its sample who had been treated for the three principal organic causes of impotence—diabetes, heart disease, and hypertension—only 23 percent of them reported that they were completely impotent. Not surprisingly, this was the same percentage of those taking the four principal medications associated with impotence (cardiac, antihypertensive, hypoglycemic, and vasodilator agents) who reported complete impotence.[59]

What can we conservatively claim may contribute to impotence? Increasing age is the factor most highly associated with impotence. In addition to the above-mentioned diseases and medications, impotence is strongly associated with psychosocial conditions, such as depression (50 to 90 percent of depressed men report decreased sexual activity) and anger—but not obesity, frequency or amount of smoking and alcohol, and sixteen of seventeen measured hormones, including testosterone, other androgens, and other sex hormones.[60]

Sexual dysfunction may also be caused by automobile, sports, and other accidents in which blunt injury to the pelvis and the perineum (the area between the base of the scrotum and the anus) occurs. Athletes are especially vulnerable to injuries such as being hit in the pelvic area by a hockey puck or baseball. Falling on the crossbar of a boy's bicycle is the most frequent trauma found to cause sports-related sexual dysfunctions. Coaches should demand protective perineal equipment be designed for their boys, especially because erectile dysfunction may delay its appearance until the boys are older.[61] Boys should ride girls' bicycles.

I don't believe that any scientifically defensible statement can be made at this stage in research about the relative contribution that organic and psychosocial causes make to impotence. Whereas using the narrower definition of impotence, as erectile deficiency, focuses attention on the most immediate biochemical and physiological mechanisms mediating impotence, using a man's more subjective judgments about his own sexual impotence and satisfaction focuses attention on a richer variety of both physical as well as psychosocial causes. This is not to deny, of course, that the latter do not alter the body's chemistry and physiology in ways that may affect potency, an understanding of which may provide insights about possible treatment protocols.

TREATMENT. The centuries-long search for elusive aphrodisiacs, such as ground-up rhinoceros horns, believed to heighten and sustain adolescent desire and pleasure, is apparently over. Thailand's English-speaking newspaper, *The Nation*, reported that an application has been sent to the FDA to approve a drug, named Libido. It is a pure freeze-dried chicken-egg extract that stimulated testosterone production in 85 percent of Norwegian men. Reflecting men's eternal hope, the drug's creators are so confident about its aphrodisiac properties, as yet to be demonstrated, that they plan to offer a two-week supply of one hundred capsules for the sexual athletes among us, at a reported cost of the equivalent of $150![62]

Why are some urologists, in particular, so confident that most impotent men can recover their erectile potency? In the words of one, there has been a "staggering" increase in understanding the biochemistry and physiology of erections,[63] which has contributed to the development of new erectile-producing drugs. Walsh and Donker's[64] classic 1982 report describing the nerve-bundle pathways that control erections heralded a flood of research on the structure and physiology of the penis, the mechanisms of relaxing the corpora cavernosum to enhance arterial inflow and the constricting of the venal outflow necessary to make the penis rigid.[65]

Another reason for the euphoric belief of some urologists that men no longer need endure the frustration, shame, and unhappiness that impotence can produce is the availability of a variety of more reliable treatment options. Each has its hopeful advocates. However, the considered judgment of the experts participating in the 1992 NIH consensus conference is that the various options' "long-term efficacy is in general relatively low. Moreover, there is a high rate of voluntary cessation of treatment for all currently popular forms of therapy for erectile dysfunction."[66]

Which option to select depends upon the reasons for the sexual dysfunction. When organic causes for impotence cannot be determined, sex education and/or counseling may be helpful alone or combined with other treatment options. Widespread ignorance by men of their own and women's bodies and sexual sensitivities and functions, age-related complications, the different meanings that sex has for men and women, and varied sexual techniques, when combined with men's reserve and inhibition to talk about sex with their partners, suggest that education be the first option to be explored. Persistent inhibitions and psychic conflicts about sex make counseling or behavior therapy targeted to deinhibiting a man's sexual responses a second option. Costs may become an issue for most if therapy continues for more than several sessions.

Whether impotence may be psychologically or organically caused, a noninvasive, relatively safe, and widely used vacuum device can produce an erection in most men. It has been available for several decades. In 1982, the FDA approved the first external vacuum device—called EricAid—for distribution with a physician's prescription by the Osbon Foundation.[67] Vacuum devices operate by inserting the penis in a plastic tube, creating a vacuum around the penis which pulls blood into the penis, filling the spaces in its corpora cavernosum so creating an erection in a few minutes. A ring is then slipped around the base of the penis to prevent the blood from flowing out and the cylinder is then removed. An erection can be sustained without pain or discomfort for about thirty minutes. The ring may impair ejaculation in some; others may find the device uncomfortable. While the Osbon Foundation claims that 90 percent of impotent men succeed in getting an erection and that restoring blood flow results in recovery of naturally spontaneous erections in some men, the NIH consensus experts report a "significant rate of patient dropout."[68]

If I had known about vacuum therapy (which my urologists did not inform me about, and which the urological literature I read also did not describe), I would have selected it as my first option. As long as the corpora cavernosum has not been injured (as occurred when I opted for an inflatable prosthesis), vacuum therapy may enhance the effects of other treatments.[69] If my prosthesis must be removed in the future due to infection or leakage, I will first try the vacuum device to learn what my remaining penile tissues can absorb before trying other treatments.

Low levels of testosterone can be replaced by testosterone therapy to enhance desire and potency, which may be why the creators of Libido believe it is ready for FDA approval though not demonstrating its effects themselves. However, testosterone's contribution to potency is not well understood,[70] and its side effects must be carefully monitored, especially if men are not in good health and are predisposed to liver, kidney, and heart disease. Since testosterone may contribute to prostatic cancer, it could be a risky way to regain an erection.[71]

Increased understanding of how central nervous system neurotransmitters such as serotonin affect sexual arousal, orgasm, and ejaculation have spurred the search for oral medications that avoid invasive surgical procedures. The FDA has approved only one oral drug—pills made from the bark of the yohimbehe tree.[72] This drug may enhance sexual desire and improve erections in some, but its side effects of nausea, dizziness, and headaches may not make it worth the cost and effort for others. Since it has not been found to be effective in more than 20 percent to 35 percent of patients—not much more than found for placebos—researchers continue to search for other, more effective, oral pharmacological agents. Trazodone is one current candidate. Prescribed as an antidepressant, some patients reported that it enhanced their sexual desire and erections, possibly, so researchers hypothesize, by increasing serotonin. A noncontrolled preliminary study of men with erectile dysfunction found that younger patients, but not smokers or those over sixty years of age, responded with increased potency.[73]

As scientific understanding of the central nervous system and erectile biology advances, might not impotent men realistically hope that noninvasive oral medications may become available soon? Like Libido? Or like an "anti-impotent" pill that the drug firm Pfizer is reportedly working on? For some, the insertable pellet that another firm, Vivus, is developing may be preferable[74] to either needle injection or oral medications.

In the meantime, Upjohn marketed in 1994 an FDA-approved self-injecting drug called Caverject.[75] Though I have found no research evidence evaluating its merits, it is based on a decade of research on several drugs, such as papaverine and prostaglandin El, which when injected into the corpora cavernosum, can increase and maintain potency for several hours.[76]

My second urologist had suggested that I volunteer to go to the hospital's laboratory for an injection into my penis whenever I wished to have an erection. Well! I was not eager to be a guinea pig for an experiment whose dosage levels, pain thresholds, and emotional effects were to be determined. Nor could I imagine myself carrying my erection around for several hours and preplanning my next loving with Maryjane hours ahead of time. Nor was I too keen to have a needle stuck into my favorite organ. Besides, knowing how stubbornly independent my former penis had been, I had doubts that it would de-cock itself within three hours. I resisted having to return to the laboratory for another shot of a drug to de-erect my priapismic cock. Apparently, my worry was not singular. Drop-out rates from experiments have been high; the reasons have not yet been clarified. Immediate or delayed pain at the needle site has been reported for some men who had a radical prostatectomy even with low doses.[77]

A 1994 critical review of drug-induced erections concluded that:

> the current state of knowledge on the effects of drugs in the central and peripheral mechanisms of libido and penile erection has been built on a complex but somewhat shaky foundation. Coupled with methodological sound research, there is a patch-work of poorly designed studies, uncontrolled trials, clinical impressions and single case reports. It is not surprising, therefore, that confusion prevails in our understanding of drugs influencing libido and erections.[78]

Despite such a gloomy assessment and since Upjohn's research passed FDA standards, I would have tried Caverject to discover its fit for me and my penis even though it cost $20 to $25 a shot—a more economical erection than my current inflatable prosthesis is costing me for Stubby II's occasional relaxation treatment.

A relatively rare cause of impotence is venous deformity, obstruction, or leakage which can be treated surgically. Diagnostic procedures are not yet reliable enough to identify which patients may benefit from the operation for both the short- and long-term. Apparently the operation helps only a minority of patients and the relapse rate is high. As for any operation, costs quickly become a limiting factor to selecting this option.[79]

Finally, erectile deficiency can be remedied by implants, which I opted for in the early eighties' dark days before urologists became excited about their discoveries of how marvelously complex an erection's mechanisms are. Though some twenty thousand men a year opt for implants, I would have experimented with other options first if I had known about them or if they had been available. Implants permanently alter the penis's corpora cavernosum and possibly nerves.[80]

Despite my diligent efforts to ferret out information about the immediate and enduring psychic effects of the treatments available, I had not anticipated their specific lingering emotional effects on my health and sexuality, which my inner doctor was telling me now to examine. But have I won a Pyrrhic victory? Is my inner doctor's increasing restlessness warning me that the changes I have made in my life may ultimately make me less healthy and happy?

The lingering effects of cancer and impotence on my relationships

My editor's request to write this epilogue impelled me to explore what my inner doctor had been urging me to do. I settled into a deeply meditative, barely conscious, mood. Suddenly a vivid but troubling dreamlike sequence of images filled me. Maryjane and I were being carried up a steep London escalator to the theater district. We were standing side-by-side, holding hands, looking up toward the theater's lights at the top. Then to my dismay the escalator split into two parallel halves. Maryjane began to move ahead of me. Our hands separated. My half began to slow down, and then it reversed its direction, moving back toward the black tube-station below. I looked down into its darkness. It was not forbidding; I was fascinated by what was there. I knew I would reach it before Maryjane reached the lights. London's subway escalators are lined by framed advertisements on each side. Maryjane's side was lined by numerous frames of familiar and unfamiliar faces. My side wasn't; many of its frames were indistinct; the majority were empty.

I had no doubts. My inner physician had reentered my life to warn me about my cancer, impotence, and current way of living. But what was she saying? My answers came too slowly to meet my editor's deadline, perhaps because I was not as emotionally vulnerable or as willing to explore her meanings in as great a depth as I had earlier. So for clues, I reread this book a second, third, and then a fourth time. I had "forgotten" many of my earlier laboriously won insights. But I encountered many of the same themes and, surprisingly, earlier intimations, warnings, and predictions that my current dream still seems to express and which have since occurred. I had no doubts. Healing the emotional effects of cancer and impotence is not yet complete.

What did her symbols mean? Togetherness and separation? Up and down? Forward and backward? Full and empty picture frames? Light and dark? And why was I only troubled, dismayed, and fascinated? Not overwhelmed, frightened, or saddened? What do these questions tell me about the mysteries of living?

Togetherness and separation

I love Maryjane as much as always; this past Christmas I promised her it was forever. But we are increasingly traveling in different directions as the dream dismayingly highlights. When separated we still talk daily on the phone; we still continue to work effortlessly as a team; we still enjoy our biannual excursions abroad; I still restlessly and intermittently hold her in my arms throughout the night; I still feel her triumphs and defeats; I still feel enormously protective of her, even though she has become a highly independent professional woman.

But we are increasingly separating both physically and emotionally from each other. Like many other two-career couples in their late middle years, we don't share as many common activities as we did when creating our family and building our homes. Our current lives are so busy that we must plan where and when to meet six months—sometimes a year—ahead to vacation together; we have too few weekends free together to entertain or be spontaneously playful.

More importantly, my routes to health are not hers. Her career is consumingly filled with people; mine no longer is. Sex is on her terms of frequent hugs and kisses but has not been on mine since the year of Stubby's arrival.

Too singularly focused on avoiding nature's stresses, I unwittingly created a way of life that I had not anticipated she would not want to share. She prefers the thermostat to be fifty-six degrees, I sixty-seven; she avoids sunlight, I seek it; she prefers cross-country skiing, I swimming laps outdoors; she doesn't care to give or receive massages, I do; she has not tried to visit me this year at my winter's retreat or remain at our summer home for as long as I do; she needs to be in frequent contact with Lucy, our grandsons, and her career's network of clients, I don't. I want to test and take advantage of what health I still have by traveling biannually to exotic third-world countries, she doesn't; I enjoy vigorous physical adventures, such as trekking, in the Far East, she doesn't.

Up and down

"Up and down" do not refer to our careers' success. Possessed by her career, she continues to go "up." She has assumed more and more responsibility at the state and national level and consulted internationally. Was I envious? Not at all. I am very proud, even awed, by how her dogged dedication to her writing, workshops, and board positions have brought her increased prominence. Furthermore, my career has not gone "down." It has taken, however, an oblique turn away from direct individual legal and personal consultations to more national involvement as a reflective elder "statesman" in my field of specialty. Bringing my feminine inner doctor more into awareness may have nourished greater creativity during my isolated months at my winter and summer retreats. The three books I have written there since 1988 have been well received.

No, "up and down," my sexy mind tells me, refers to Stubby II's retirement from sex with Maryjane—the "downer" I had feared might occur. While satisfyingly "up" for Maryjane, he was not satisfying me. Though just as sexy as always, I, somewhat perversely, was pleased to learn I was different. The majority of men in one pioneering study of their quality of life reported they did not feel sexy after their treatment: 58 percent reported decreased sexual interest and 74 percent decreased sexual enjoyment.[81] But Stubby's increasing failure to evoke my orgasm after 568 days undermined Maryjane's feelings of adequacy. As other men have reported to sex counselors also, Stubby's decreased sensitivity required much more direct and vigorous stimulation than she was emotionally willing to give. While not technologically impotent, I became emotionally so when relying on only our typical ways of loving. After months of abortive efforts to reclaim my orgasms, she eventually said, "I don't want any more sex." Not unexpectedly, research shows that impotence precipitously occurs with increasing frustration with one's sex life and partner.[82] Spouses not only report greater worry, tenseness, and general distress than men about their illness—but also reduced sexual interest and enjoyment as well.[83]

Aware, from my former divorce work, that happily married couples mutually enjoy sex and unhappily married ones certainly don't, how could I sustain my love by separating it from my insistent need for sex? Though I had sensed when first getting Stubby that Maryjane might not be as responsive as he would need her to be, I hadn't thought through what I would do if she weren't.

Only now in retrospect do I understand how I have unconsciously severely squelched my sexual desire for her since and how subtly that has affected the way I relate and don't want to relate to her. Hugs yes; kisses on her cheeks, yes. Holding her clothed breasts, yes. What she wants and continues to ask for, yes. I strongly need to touch and feel physically close to another; I'll be an erotically touching skin-to-skin person until I die.

I now no longer feel an urge to have sex with Maryjane. I no longer have "the subconscious of a cock when . . . around her." A whiff of sexual arousal is so painful that I unconsciously avoid it. Just as I had averted my eyes *not* to see young bucks with bulging crotches walking down the street when I couldn't face the loss of my cock, so now I don't want to see her naked or feel her naked in bed, which she hasn't been for years. Or, like a pubertal boy uncomfortable about what to do with his emerging sexuality, I now uncontrollably squirm and close my eyes when I see a man making love to—even just kissing—a woman in a movie. I no longer feel good glancing at young women in their disappearing bikinis languorously stretched out along my condo's pool, nor do I easily talk with Maryjane about sex, which I had unconsciously sealed off from our conversations. I no longer make the corny sexual jokes or sexy play on words that I used to. When I last tried to, Maryjane exploded. With tongue in cheek, I said I might write an article, for a law journal, arguing that the enticing nudity of young women's disappearing bikinis was sexual harassment of voyeuristic but vulnerable men not able to control their erections. "They should learn to control them," my feminist wife insisted. Easier for a woman to say than for a man to do. Why haven't nuns gotten into as much sexual trouble as monks and priests have?

Such severe repression of my sexual desire for Maryjane and its unnecessary, even inappropriate, extension to other women now tells me how intensely frustrated I have been—and how much energy I have been consuming to protect myself from its arousal. My impotence with her and feelings of incompleteness have disconnected us at the very core of my sexual being. Just as the loss of spontaneous erections risked emotionally thinning my relationships, so loss of sexual desire, spilling over to dampen my erotic playfulness, is muting the emotional richness of our former relationship. I had thought both might occur if I did *not* get my erections back; I had not really anticipated their lingering severity *after* I had.

Not until I read Schover's comments about what men tell sex counselors did I realize how typical my reactions have been.

> When erectile dysfunction occurs after cancer treatment, many men stop initiating lovemaking. They dread being unable to have an erection, both in terms of their own self-esteem and their partner's disappointment. [Not relevant to Stubby or me but lovemaking's frustration is.] Unfortunately, most men do not voice these feelings, leaving partners to surmise that the patient no longer desires sex, or more specifically, is no longer interested in them. The decreased sexual activity often is accompanied by a decline in the expression of nonsexual affection. The husband fears that his wife will interpret a hug or a pat as a sexual advance.[84]

Given the centrality of sex to my feelings of maleness, what was I to do to keep my desire, orgasmic potential, and Stubby's alive? As I wrote in Chapter 7 when discovering my erotic nature, to feel sexually primed is to feel alive; to have no desire is to be dead—an emotional equation with which I have lived subconsciously since Old Faithful reared his head.

Forward and backward

Maryjane's escalator kept going forward; mine was beginning to reverse. Why did mine not continue forward with her, even though on a separate track? Forward to where?

A mistress? No. Separation from Maryjane does not mean connecting with other women—repression of my sexual desire for scantily clad young women reaffirms that. For me, a mistress has always risked the dangerous transformation of sexual fulfillment into love. Faithfulness to Maryjane is too integral to my character.

A gay partner? No. Maryjane is my life-long partner. I have not yet thought of myself as gay. I have not discovered any gay "life style" with which I feel at home; nor do I feel accepted at gay bars and churches, gay men's workshops, or other such groups that I have explored to test that possibility. Might my commitment to her be preventing me from fulfilling an intensifying adolescent desire for a close intimate male friendship? Might such a relationship sap the vitality of my love for her? While I've not tested that thought, I've been wondering if my increasing sexual vulnerability could impel me to.

Celibacy? No! If I can't control my appetite for gravy and whipped cream, how can I expect to suppress Stubby II's needs without heightening my body's tenseness and incurring frustrated resentment? Feeling sexy is too central to my feeling alive. Besides, would my Stubbys have been for naught?

Masturbation? No. If my escalator had stopped when it split, then perhaps that would be the way to separate love for Maryjane from my need for sex. While always necessary and available, the dream says it is not the direction my inner doctor is pointing toward. Why? As I have written, sex for me has always meant connecting with others. The growing solitariness of my ways of coping healthily with nature's stress and my body's needs, which encourage masturbation, may, paradoxically, be hastening my death. While perhaps an emotionally exaggerated view, isolation from intimate enduring relationships with others, as occurs in bachelors and widowed men and from the community of others, as research has also shown,[85] can lead to illness and early death.

My inner doctor reversed the escalator's direction. Why? Did "backward" mean turning from the third back to the second revelation—communion with males, a communion I had had sporadic experiences of since 1988? Or did it mean reencountering and really transcending the mystery of dying and its associated darkness and blackness? Or both?

Maryjane says retreating to the pubertal sources of my communion with males is, in the words of psychoanalysts, "regressing in the service of the ego to an earlier fixation point." Damn! Regression can lead to completing earlier experiences whose unfulfillment has blocked, or messed up, subsequent development. Regression or not, my happiest postcancer and postimpotence experiences have been with two male friends.

While on my first business trip back to the Philippines where Juan's ministry cured my depression in 1983, I met two young men whose friendship showed me a different way of relating to males: Manuel, a twenty-nine-year-old married masseur, and Andy, a thirty-two-year-old American wanderer, who obsessively talked about bedding one woman after another. Both taught me that men could be spontaneously and physically affectionate, "emotional, utterly open, even wild[ly], erotic" with each other. Andy was so naturally affectionate that he was not aware how frequently he put his arm around or hugged me, even in American grocery stores or on New Delhi's streets; Manuel would spontaneously take my hand when we hiked with his married friends who were similarly demonstrative. Each became my playful traveling companion as I explored the Far East every fall and spring: whitewater rafting in India's mountainous Darjeeling region, living on a Kashmir houseboat, keeping each other warm at 14,000 feet in a small pup tent on one of Pakistan's remote trails when an unexpected November snowstorm whipped through our thin jackets, riding an elephant to visit a smokey and darkly mysterious Thailand opium den, being massaged in an illegal gay Hong Kong steam bath, cowering behind a large jungle tree to keep out of sight of a charging Nepalese rhinoceros, hiking through northern Luzon and exploring its beaches with Manuel's prankish and playful gang of infrequently employed friends desperate for the money I paid them to support their families.

What about sex? Sex was neither Andy's nor Manuel's and his gang's way with other males. In contrast to Juan, Manuel rarely massaged my Stubby. I never asked him to do so. But the erotic was their way—most prominently in Manuel's and our gang's playfulness—seeing sex everywhere and in everything, joking about it, affectionately roughhousing, touching, hugging, leaning on and holding each other's hands, playfully grabbing each other's crotches; questioning me about sex with Maryjane and the size of my cock; teaching me their native dialect words to greet others on the trail, which I innocently did to their hilarious outbursts (they had taught me their slang words for sexual invitations); bathing and playfully splashing each other in mountain streams after a hard day's climb, and swimming nude in coastal green-blue waters. Such experiences bonded us together in the kind of natural, mutually accepting, and adventuresome fraternity that I had begun to have when I was an adolescent before moving away. They helped me recover and relive communion's pubertal meanings. I have felt what it is to be a whole person, to be my natural, uninhibited erotic *male* self. I have been celebrating my maleness these past eight years.

As I explored and fulfilled my incompleted adolescent potentials and became the young man I could have been, I was finally able to let Pete go emotionally. He no longer is a symbol of the youthful desires and dreams I had never fulfilled when younger. I don't sense, however, that he has let me go.

Full and empty picture frames

My immersion in my solitary writing way of life hid from me the fact that many of my escalator's framed pictures had become vaguer and emptier which my dream compelled me now to acknowledge. Only two of my pictured male friends have remained youthful enough in heart that I would want to spend time with them. The others are rather stodgy and stuffy; besides, we are too busy to keep in touch. Resigning from my firm and not taking on new clients (thus freeing myself to write uninterruptedly), wintering in Mexico (where my fleeting command of the local language is not sufficient for me to know others well), summering for months on an isolated part of the seacoast, giving up some of my board and committee work because of too frequent absences, traveling extensively during the fall and spring, emotionally letting Pete go but not yet forming an easy and open adult relationship with him, seeing Lucy and my grandchildren only occasionally, and increasing separations from Maryjane—all of these isolating experiences are emotionally blurring and emptying too many frames.

Andy's frame is also becoming vaguer. Consumed by his work and love for a woman abroad whom he now visits whenever free, we seldom see or travel with each other. Manuel's frame has recently become empty. For years he begged me to loan him funds to build a house for his wife and child. When I did, he used the money instead to leave his family to emigrate illegally to America. When I last saw him I told him he had betrayed my trust—the foundation for any real friendship.

It is too soon to tell if I have now transcended my need for such playful "gang" experiences and am ready to connect differently with men in the future. However, being too much alone and my increasing loneliness are making me depressed. Is my inner doctor telling me that too many empty frames are unhealthy?

Cancer's and impotence's challenge to the mysteries of living

Light and darkness

For me, light is life, darkness is death. Cancer's possible recurrence, compounded by the beginning of aging's loss of dependable bodily control, means I live more consciously with my mortality. I know dying a little more intimately now; the phrase from the Twenty-third Psalm, "Though I walk through the valley of the shadow of death," enters my mind more frequently.

Why am I not overwhelmed, frightened, or saddened by the escalator's beginning reversal? I am only troubled and dismayed—though fascinated—by moving toward the underground's darkness. When I first learned I had cancer, I wanted to have "six or seven more years to digest, reflect, translate, express what I had learned." Having had those years has brought a greater emotional acceptance of, even serenity about, dying. I now occasionally look forward to encountering its mystery. I feel I have had my reprieve; more years now are like dessert—delightful but not so indispensable.

I have even begun to look back to my cancer with friendlier eyes. It compelled me to turn deeply inward, to know myself better; I discovered my inner doctor; I took my life more into my own hands to reorder my priorities; I've traveled to places and had adventures with Andy and Manuel that I probably never would have had if I had continued my former way of life; I am more prepared now for future illness and death. Cancer now no longer frightens me. Nor does death; I've cleared, so to speak, more of my emotional decks for its entrance.

Transcendence and resurrection

But my inner physician keeps saying, "Not yet! Not yet!" Her reentrance into my life tells me she believes there are new opportunities for more growth as I move toward death's underground. Paradoxically transcending my fears of death frees me to live more fully—scarcely a novel insight to most religions. One sign of my transcendence is my growing freedom from my self-centered pursuit of my body's health. Now that cancer's return is less likely, why not now yield more to, and test how well I can adapt to, nature's stresses? My interpersonal—not my body's—health is the way to live more fully, even if at the expense of my body's serenity. So I am stepping over to Maryjane's escalator by selling my Mexican time-shares and reducing the amount of time I spend at our summer home separated from her.

"Not yet! Not yet!" also tells me I need another six to seven years; my wily inner physician has found three more books for me to write—but where Maryjane is. I can buy a space heater!

Are my loneliness and depression about losing Andy, Manuel, and our gang telling me that I need to find other faces to fill those empty escalator frames? But where to find other companions as erotically playful and affectionately demonstrative to travel the world with, which I still long to do?

What is to happen to Stubby II, the central character of my last chapter, "A Golden Resurrection"? He was my means to becoming an "adventurous, playful, erotic, expressive, exciting" male—to feeling alive, which sex has always meant to me. He was my technological route to wholeness. The unexpected irony is that I have him but now don't know what to do with him. Until aging's decreasing testosterone and other vicissitudes diminish his recurringly intense desires, his availability will disturb and test me again and again.

I now have intimations that I may have subconsciously lied to myself about the meaning of wholeness when I wrote that "God was the given organizing spirit and principle of wholeness for which my inner physician had been the agent." Is ultimate transcendence my free choice no longer to proudly raise up Stubby II? Is that what resurrection is to mean for me? To freely give up my dogma that sexiness is aliveness and to discover and accept God's meaning of wholeness?

Notes

Preface

1. L. R. Schover, "Sexual Rehabilitation after Treatment for Prostate Cancer," *Cancer* 71 (1993): 1024–30.

2. G. Kolata, "Prostate Cancer Consensus Hampered by Lack of Data," *Science* 236 (1987): 1626–27.

3. J. O'C. Hamilton, "Milken vs. Cancer," *Business Week* (January 9, 1995): 36–37.

4. H. I. Scher, "Introduction: Prostate Cancer," *Seminars in Oncology* 21 (1944): 511–13.

5. I. M. Thompson, et al., "An Opportunity to Determine Optimal Treatment of pT3 Prostate Cancer: The Window May Be Closing," *Urology* 44 (1994): 804–11.

6. G. L. Andriole, "Editorial: Prostate Cancer," *The Journal of Urology* 154 (1995): 1102,

7. R. Thomas, "Editorial: The Evolving World of Urological Laparoscopy," *The Journal of Urology* 154 (1995): 487–88.

8. F. J. Fowler, Jr., et al., "Patient-Reported Complications and Follow-Up Treatment after Radical Prostatectomy," *Urology* 42 (1993): 622–29; G. W. Jones, "Magnitude of the Problem: American College of Surgeons Database and Epidemiologic Study," *Cancer* 71 (1993): 887–90; R. A. Morton, Jr., "Racial Differences in Adenocarcinoma of the Prostate in North American Men," *Urology* 44 (1994): 637–45.

9. W. J. Catalona, "Screening for Prostate Cancer: Enthusiasm," *Urology* 42 (1993): 113–15; Jones, 1993.

10. D. S. Coffey, "Prostate Cancer. An Overview of an Increasing Dilemma," *Cancer Supplement* 71 (1993); J. A. Freeman, et al., "Adjuvant Radiation, Chemotherapy, and Androgen Deprivation Therapy for Pathologic Stage D1 Adenocarcinoma of the Prostate," *Urology* 44 (1994): 719–25; J. Marx, "New Clue to Prostate Cancer Spread," *Science* 268 (1995): 799–800;

an ABC News, "Good Morning America" (May 22, 1996) broadcast reported the higher estimate.

11. Morton, 1994.

12. P. C. Walsh, "Prostate Cancer Kills: Strategy to Reduce Deaths," *Urology* 44 (1994a): 463–66.

13. M. K. Brawer, "Editorial: Prostate Cancer Detection," *The Journal of Urology* 151 (1994): 1308–1309; Catalona, 1993; J. B. deKernion, "Editorial: Prostate Cancer," *The Journal of Urology* 150 (1993): 390; Freeman, et al., 1994; R. G. Middleton, "Editorial: Prostate Cancer," *The Journal of Urology* 151 (1994): 655.

14. P. H. Lange, "Controversies in Management of Apparently Localized Carcinoma of Prostate," *Supplement to Urology* 34 (1989): 13–18; P. C. Walsh, "Radical Prostatectomy: A Procedure in Evolution," *Seminars in Oncology* 21, (1994b): 662–71.

15. F. C. da Silva, "Quality of Life in Prostatic Cancer Patients," *Cancer* 72 (1993): 3803–3806; F. C. da Silva, et al., "Quality of Life in Patients with Prostatic Cancer," *Cancer* 71 (1993): 1138–42; S. D. Fossa, N. Aass, and S. Opjordsmoen, "Assessment of Quality of Life in Patients with Prostate Cancer," *Seminars in Oncology* 21 (1994): 657–61; A.B. Kornblith, et al., "Quality of Life of Patients with Prostate Cancer and Their Spouses," *Cancer* 73 (1994): 2791–2802; Schover, 1993; J. W. Sharp, "Expanding the Definition of Quality of Life for Prostate Cancer," *Cancer* 71 (1993): 1078–82

16. *Honolulu Star Bulletin,* November 21, 1995, A–6.

17. W. Bihrle, III, "Editorial: Impotence: Expanding the Horizons," *The Journal of Urology* 153 (1995): 1139; A. Morales, "Editorial: Impotence," *The Journal of Urology* 151 (1994): 1238; Schover, 1993.

18. National Library of Medicine, U.S. Department of Health & Human Services, "Impotence," *Current Bibliographies in Medicine,* 1992, No. 92–8, 40 pp.

19. H A. Feldman, et al., "Impotence and Its Medical and Psychosocial Correlates: Results of the Massachusetts Male Aging Study," *The Journal of Urology* 151 (1994): 54–61.

Chapter 1

1. B. Rollin, *First, You Cry* (New York: Harper & Row, 1976).

2. C. A. Oisson, "Staging Lymphadenectomy Should be an Antecedent to Treatment in Localized Prostatic Carcinoma," *Supplement to Urology* 25, no. 2 (1985): 4–6.

3. J. D. Schmidt, et al., "Trends in Patterns of Care for Prostatic Cancer,

1974–1983: Results of Surveys by the American College of Surgeons," *The Journal of Urology* 136 (1986): 416–21.

4. C. A. Olsson, R. Babazan, and R. V. White, "Surgical Management of Stage B or C Prostatic Carcinoma: Radical Surgery vs. Radiotherapy," *Supplement to Urology* 25, no. 2 (1985): 30–35.

5. Ibid.

6. M. V. Pilepich, et al., "Radical Prostatectomy or Radiotherapy in Carcinoma of Prostate: The Dilemma Continues," *Urology* 30 (1987): 18–21.

7. Kolata, 1987.

Chapter 2

1. J. L. Marx, "The Immune System 'Belongs in the Body,' " *Science* 227 (March 8, 1985): 1190–92.

2. Olsson, et al., 1985.

Chapter 4

1. N. Cousins, *Saturday Review* (October 1, 1977): 16.

2. N. Cousins, *Anatomy of an Illness as Perceived by the Patient* (New York: W. W. Norton, 1979).

Chapter 5

1. Cousins, 1979, p. 159.

2. Schmidt, et al., 1986.

3. G. Kolata, "Is the War on Cancer Being Won?" *Science* 229 (1985): 543–44.

4. H. Bush, "Cancer: The New Synthesis," *Science* 84 (1984): 34–39; Kolata, 1985.

5. Bush, 1984, p. 35.

6. A. J. Sattilaro, *Recalled by Life* (Boston: Houghton Mifflin Co., 1982); A. J. Sattilaro and T. Monte, *Living Well Naturally* (Boston: Houghton Mifflin Co., 1984).

7. C. B. Simone, *Cancer and Nutrition* (New York: McGraw-Hill Book Co., 1983), p. xii.

8. C. B. Thomas, K. R. Duszynski, and J. W. Shaffer, "Family Attitudes Reported in Youth as Potential Predictors of Cancer," *Psychosomatic Medicine* 41 (1979): 287–302.

9. L. LeShan, *You Can Fight for Your Life. Emotional Factors in the Treatment of Cancer* (New York: M. Evans & Co., 1977).

Chapter 6

1. E. Mukamel, J. Hanna, and J. B. de Kernion, "Pitfalls in Preoperative Staging in Prostate Cancer," *Urology* 30 (1987): 318–21; P. Ray, et al., "Staging Errors in Prostatic Cancer," *The Journal of Urology* 132 (1984): 1125–26; I. M. Thompson, et al., "Adenocarcinoma of the Prostate: Results of Routine Urological Screening," *The Journal of Urology* 132 (1984): 690–92.

2. R. R. Bahnson, J. E. Garnett, and J. T. Grayhack, "Adjuvant Radiation Therapy in Stages C and D1 Prostatic Adenocarcinoma," *Urology* 27 (1986): 403–406; R. P. Gibbons, et al., "Adjuvant Radiotherapy Following Radical Prostatectomy: Results and Complications," *The Journal of Urology* 135 (1986): 65–68; M. Golimbu, J. Provet, S. Al-Askari, and P. Morales, "Radical Prostatectomy for Stage D1 Prostate Cancer," *Urology* 30 (1987): 427–35; P. H. Lange, et al., "Radiation Therapy as Adjuvant Treatment after Radical Prostatectomy: Patient Tolerance and Preliminary Results," *The Journal of Urology* 136 (1986): 45–49; G. R. Ray, M. A. Bagshaw, and F. Freiha, "External Beam Radiation Salvage for Residual or Recurrent Local Tumor Following Radical Prostatectomy," *The Journal of Urology* 132 (1984): 926–30.

Chapter 7

1. S. Hite, *The Hite Report on Male Sexuality* (New York: Alfred Knopf, 1981).

2. S. J. Silber, *The Male: A Comprehensive and Clearly Written Guide to the Male Sexual System* (New York: Charles Scribner's Sons, 1981).

3. R. Milsten, *Male Sexual Function: Myth, Fantasy, and Reality* (New York: Avon Books, 1979), pp. 20–21.

4. R. and E. MacKenzie, *New York Times,* June 24, 1984. The headquarters of Impotence Anonymous is located at 119 South Ruth Street, Maryville, TN 37801–5798.

5. Hite, 1981, pp. 390, 395.

6. P. C. Walsh and P. J. Donker, "Impotence Following Radical Prostatectomy: Insight into Etiology and Prevention," *The Journal of Urology* (1982): 492–97.

7. I. D. Sharlip and W. L. Furlow, "Overview of International Society for Impotence Research," *Urology* 30 (1987): 205–208.

Chapter 8

1. Rollin, 1976.
2. T. Vanggaard, *Phallos: A Symbol and Its History in the Male World.* Reprint (New York: International Universities Press, Inc., 1974).
3. Ibid., p. 18.
4. Ibid., p. 74.

Chapter 9

1. Hite, 1981, p. 608.
2. Ibid., p. 615.
3. Ibid., p. 555.
4. E. D. Whitehead and E. Leiter, "New Frontiers in Alloplastic Genitourinary Prostheses. II. The Surgical Management of Erectile Impotence," *New York State Journal of Medicine* (December 1982): 1806–11.
5. I. J. Fishman, F. B. Scott, and J. K. Light, "Experience with Inflatable Penile Prosthesis," special issue to *Urology* 23 (1984): 86–92; M. C. S. Googe and T. M. Mook, "The Inflatable Penile Prosthesis: New Developments," *American Journal of Nursing,* (1983): 1044–47; D. C. Merrill, "Mentor Inflatable Penile Prosthesis: Clinical Experience in 52 Patients," *British Association of Urological Surgeons* 56 (1984): 512–15; D. C. Merrill and P. Javaheri, "Mentor Inflatable Penile Prosthesis: Preliminary Clinical Results in 30 Patients," special issue to *Urology* 23 (1984): 72–74.
6. R. C. Benson, D. M. Barrett, and D. E. Patterson, "The Jonas Prosthesis-Technical Considerations and Results," *The Journal of Urology* 130 (1983): 920–22; D. K. Montague, "Experience with Jonas Malleable Penile Prosthesis," special issue to *Urology* 23 (1984): 83–85.
7. D. C. Merrill, "Clinical Experience with Mentor Inflatable Penile Prosthesis in 206 Patients," *Urology* 28 (1986): 185–89.
8. L. E. Beutler, et al., "Women's Satisfaction with Their Partners' Penile Implants: Inflatable vs. Noninflatable Prostheses," *Urology* (1984): 552–58.
9. L. E. Beutler, et al., "Inflatable and Noninflatable Penile Prostheses: Comparative Follow-up Evaluation," *Urology* 27 (1986): 136–43; K. E. Schlamowitz, et al., "Reactions to the Implantation of an Inflatable Penile Prosthesis Among Psychogenically and Organically Impotent Men," *The Journal of Urology* 129 (1983): 295–98.

Chapter 10

1. L. Shapero and A. A. Goodman, *Never Say Die: A Doctor and Patient Talk About Breast Cancer* (New York: Appleton-Century-Crofts, 1980).
2. R. P. Gibbons, et al., "Total Prostatectomy for Localized Prostatic Cancer," *The Journal of Urology* 131 (1984): 73–76.
3. R. C. Benson, Jr., et al., "Bilateral Pelvic Lymphadenectomy and Radical Retropubic Prostatectomy for Adenocarcinoma Confined to the Prostate," *The Journal of Urology* 131 (1984): 1103–1106.
4. C. Turkington, "Disfigured Need Help for Inner Wounds," *Monitor* (American Psychological Association, July 6–7, 1984): 6.

Chapter 11

1. J. Durden-Smith, "Male and Female—Why?" *The Collegiate Career Woman* (Winter 1980–81): 9–18.

Chapter 12

1. Hite, 1981, p. 552.
2. Ibid., p. 600.

Epilogue

1. E.S. Geary, et al., "Nerve Sparing Radical Prostatectomy: A Different View," *The Journal of Urology* 154 (1995): 145–49; Schover, 1993.
2. J. Adolfsson, G. Steineck, and W. F. Whitmore, Jr., "Recent Results of Management of Palpable Clinically Localized Prostate Cancer," *Cancer* 72 (1993): 310–22; Thompson, et al., 1994; P. C. Walsh, 1994b.
3. Adolfsson, et al., 1993; Coffey, 1993; Lange, 1989; Schover, 1993; P. H. Smith and M. K. B. Parmar, "Adjuvant Therapy in Prostatic Cancer," *Cancer Supplement* 71 (1993): 992–95; Walsh, 1994b; Walsh and Donker, 1982.
4. Thompson, et al., 1994.
5 R. P. Meyers, "Editorial: Prostate Cancer—Neurovascular Preservation; Smoking Cessation May Enhance Prognosis?" *The Journal of Urology* 154 (1995): 158–59; P. E. Zimmern, J. Kaswick, and G. E. Leach, *The Journal of Urology* 154 (1955): 1110.
6. Lange, 1989.

7. Smith, Jr., J. A. "Commentary on the Desired Tissue Effects for Laser Treatment of the Prostate and How They Can Best Be Achieved?" *The Journal of Urology* 153 (1995): 2.

8. I. S. Gill, R. V. Clayman, and E. M. McDougall, "Advances in Urological Laparoscopy," *The Journal of Urology* 154 (1995): 1275–94; D. A. Levy and M. I. Resnick, "Laparoscopic Pelvic Lymphadenectomy and Radical Perineal Prostatectomy: A Viable Alternative to Radical Retropubic Prostatectomy," *The Journal of Urology* 151 (1994): 905–908.

9. Adolfsson, et al., 1993; C. B. Brendler, "Editorial: Prostate Cancer," *The Journal of Urology* 150 (1993): 1865–66; C. W. S. Cheng, E. J. Bergstrath, and H. Zincke, "Stage D1 Prostate Cancer," *Cancer* 71 (1993): 996–1004; Lange, 1989.

10. P. H. Smith, et al., 1993; A. D. Steinfeld, "Questions Regarding the Treatment of Localized Prostate Cancer," *Radiology* 184 (1992): 593–98; Thompson, et al., 1994; A. L. Zeitman, W. U. Shipley, and C. G. Willett, "Residual Disease after Radical Surgery or Radiation Therapy for Prostate Cancer," *Cancer* 71 (1993): 959–69.

11. S. A. Leibel, et al., "The Biological Basis and Clinical Application of Three-Dimensional Conformal External Beam Radiation Therapy in Carcinoma of the Prostate," *Seminars in Oncology* 21 (1994): 580–97; C. A. Perez, et al., "Localized Carcinoma of the Prostate (Stages T1B, T1C, T2, and T3)," *Cancer* 72 (1993): 3156–73.

12. M. A. Bagshaw, I. D. Kaplan, and R. C. Cox, "Radiation Therapy for Localized Disease," *Cancer* 71 (1993): 939–52.

13. Andriole, 1995.

14. Zeitman, et al., 1993.

15. Lange, 1989.

16. Ibid.; J. A. Freeman, et al., 1994.

17. J. B. de Kernion, 1993; A. Eisbruch, et al., "Adjuvant Irradiation after Prostatectomy for Carcinoma of the Prostate with Positive Surgical Margins," *Cancer* 73 (1994): 384–87; Thompson, et al., 1994.

18. A. J. Lim, et al., "Quality of Life: Radical Prostatectomy Versus Radiation Therapy for Prostate Cancer," *The Journal of Urology* 154 (1995): 1420–25.

19. Thompson, et al., 1994; Middleton, 1994.

20. P. R. Carroll, "Editorial: Prostate Cancer—Many Treatments but Not Enough Answers," *The Journal of Urology* 154 (1995): 454–55; J. E. Fowler, Jr., et al., "Prostate Specific Antigen after Gonadal Androgen Withdrawal and Deferred Flutamide Treatment," *The Journal of Urology* 154 (1995): 448–53; M. S. Soloway, et al., "Randomized Prospective Study Comparing Radical

Prostatectomy Alone Versus Radical Prostatectomy Preceded by Androgen Blockade in Clinical Stage B2 (T2bNx\MO) Prostate Cancer," *The Journal of Urology* 154 (1995): 424–25.

21. J. Wieder, et al., "Transrectal Ultrasound-Guided Transperineal Cryoablation in the Treatment of Prostate Carcinoma: Preliminary Results," *The Journal of Urology* 154 (1995): 435–41.

22. Gill, et al., 1995; Thomas, 1995.

23. Ibid.

24. S. C. Campbell, et al., "Open Pelvic Lymph Node Dissection for Prostate Cancer: A Reassessment," *Urology* 46 (1995): 352–55; Gill, et al., 1995.

25. D. S. Smith and W. J. Catalona, "Interexaminer Variability of Digital Rectal Examination in Detecting Prostate Cancer," *Urology* 45 (1995): 70–74; Steinfeld, 1992.

26. Catalona, 1993.

27. H. B. Carter, et al., "Nonpalable Prostate Cancer: Detection with MR Imaging," *Radiology* 178 (1991): 523–25; F. Lee, Jr., et al., "Nonpalable Cancer of the Prostate: Assessment with Transrectal US," *Radiology* 178 (1991): 197–99; Smith and Catalona, 1995; Steinfeld, 1992.

28. M. L. Blute, "Editorial: Refining the Early Detection and Staging of Prostate Cancer," *The Journal of Urology* 154 (1995): 1401–1402; Brawer, 1994; Brendler, 1993; Carter, et al., 1991; W. J. Catalona, 1993; G. W. Chodak, "Questioning the Value of Screening for Prostate Cancer in Asymptomatic Men," *Urology* 42 (1993): 116–18; de Kernion, 1993; J. E. Fowler, et al., 1995.

29. Catalona, 1993, p. 113; C. Mettlin, et al. "American Cancer Society–National Prostate Detection Project," *Cancer* 71 (1993): 891–98; M. K. Terris, et al., "Prediction of Prostate Cancer Volume Using Prostate-Specific Antigen Levels, Transrectal Ultrasound, and Systematic Sextant Biopsies," *Urology* 45 (1995): 75–80.

30. Blute, 1995; J. N. Kabalin, et al., "Serum Prostate-Specific Antigen and the Biologic Progression of Prostate Cancer," *Urology* 46 (1995): 65–70.

31. Catalona, 1993.

32. M. G. Sanda, et al., "Demonstration of a Rational Strategy for Human Prostate Cancer Gene Therapy," *The Journal of Urology* 151 (1994): 622–28.

33. Brawer, 1994

34. Marx, 1995

35. E. A. Klein, "Editorial: Prostate Cancer," *The Journal of Urology* 154 (1995): 143–44.

36. J. M. Clash, "Prostate Update," *Forbes* (October 9, 1995).

37. Walsh and Donker, 1982; P. C. Walsh, H. Lepor, and J. C. Eggleston,

83. Kornblith, et al., 1994.

84. Schover, 1993, p. 1028.

85. J. S. House, K. R. Landers, and D. Umberson, "Social Relationships and Health," *Science* 241 (1988): 540–45.